Handbook of Equine C

Handbook of Equine Colic

N. A. White II DVM MS Diplomate ACVS

Theodora Ayer Randolph Professor of Surgery, Marion duPont Scott Equine Medical Center,
VMRCVM-Virginia Tech, Leesburg, Virginia

and

G. B. Edwards BVSC DvetMed FRCVS

Professor of Equine Studies, Department of Veterinary Clinical Science and Animal Husbandry,
University of Liverpool, UK

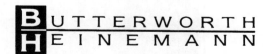

OXFORD   AUCKLAND   BOSTON   JOHANNESBURG   MELBOURNE   NEW DELHI

Butterworth-Heinemann
Linacre House, Jordan Hill, Oxford OX2 8DP
225 Wildwood Avenue, Woburn, MA 01801-2041
A division of Reed Educational and Professional Publishing Ltd

ℛ A member of the Reed Elsevier plc group

First published 1999

© Reed Educational and Professional Publishing Ltd 1999

British Library Cataloguing in Publication Data
White, Nathaniel A.
    Handbook of equine colic
    1. Colic in horses
    I.   Title II.   Edwards, G. B.
    636.1'089755

Library of Congress Cataloguing in Publication Data
White, N. A. (Nathaniel A.)
    Handbook of equine colic/N. A. White II and G. B. Edwards
    p. cm.
    Includes bibliographical references and index.
    ISBN 0 7506 3587 8
    1   Colic in horses.   I   Edwards, G. B.   II   Title.
SF959.C6W55
636.1'089755–dc21   99–35352
                                                            CIP

ISBN 0 7506 3587 8

Typeset by E & M Graphics, Midsomer Norton, Bath

Printed and bound in Great Britain by The Bath Press, Somerset

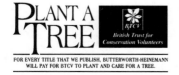

FOR EVERY TITLE THAT WE PUBLISH, BUTTERWORTH-HEINEMANN
WILL PAY FOR BTCV TO PLANT AND CARE FOR A TREE.

Contents

Preface

Veterinarians and horse owners commonly view colic as a common and inevitable disease of horses. Some have said, 'As long as there are horses we will always treat colic'. Colic also means different things to different people. To a horse owner it is often the simple abdominal disturbance easily treated by the veterinarian or a problem that might even go away with a little walking. To others, including veterinarians, colic can mean a life threatening disease. In fact, as a group, diseases that cause colic kill more horses than any other disease or group of diseases, including old age. The increased risk appears to be due to both intestinal anatomy and human management practices that favour intestinal dysfunction, impaction and mal-position more than in other animals.

The design of the equine intestine also makes diagnosis of equine intestinal diseases difficult. Most of the intestinal tract is out of reach during rectal palpation. Though the physical examination and some laboratory values are helpful, they are not specific, and the veterinarian frequently can't make a specific diagnosis and is left to treat symptoms. The signs of colic are often similar for both simple and life-threatening diseases, and the clinical signs change during the course of the disease making assessment and prognostication difficult. The dilemma of deciding which horse with colic requires surgery remains one of the greatest diagnostic challenges.

Treatments have advanced over the last 30 years as use of new analgesics and fluid therapy has improved the recovery from ileus and impaction. Veterinarians have learned that monitoring the response to treatment is a valuable tool in helping to recognize the more serious diseases. Horse owners have learned that colic means 'emergency', thereby allowing early diagnosis and treatment, and resulting in more horses surviving serious intestinal disease.

Although there are still large gaps in our knowledge about equine colic and gastrointestinal function and dysfunction, the available information makes a considerable volume of literature. The genesis of this handbook is the result of paring down the information about colic to that which is needed by the practitioner and student to examine, diagnose, treat and manage horses with colic. Prevention, though still being defined, is also included. Surgical techniques and a detailed description of surgical diseases have not been included as this information goes beyond the needs of diagnosing, treating, and preventing the most common forms of colic. We hope that this book will be of help to all those who are compelled to answer the emergency call for the horse with colic. Hopefully the information here will soon become dated with the advent of newer and better information helping to prevent the diseases that cause colic. Perhaps, eventually, we can change the perception that veterinarians will always treat colic.

Definition and causes of colic

Definition

Colic is defined as abdominal pain; specifically, pain from spasm of the colon. In the horse, the term is used to define a symptom commonly resulting from intestinal ileus or inflammation. There are numerous body movements and postures associated with colic. In a recent study by Tinker *et al* (1997), the signs and their relative frequency were recorded. The results can be seen in Table 1.1.

Incidence and mortality

The incidence of colic in the normal population is reported to range from 10–36 per cent per year (Rollins and Clement, 1979; Tinker *et al*, 1997; Uhlinger, 1992). Of these cases, approximately 80 per cent will be mild episodes where a specific diagnosis is not made, another 10 per cent are likely to be cases of impaction, flatulence or enteritis, which are diagnosed and treated successfully, and 1–2 per cent will have a serious disease, such as strangulated intestines, which requires surgery. In most cases, a specific diagnosis is never made. In a study of a normal horse population, the breakdown of diseases was approximately as follows (Tinker *et al*, 1997):

Mild idiopathic colic	83 per cent
Impaction	7 per cent
Gas colic/spasmodic	4 per cent
Gastric rupture	2 per cent
Enteritis	1 per cent
Strangulation	3 per cent

In cases of colic in a normal population of horses the mortality is less than 1 per cent (Tinker *et al*, 1997). The fatality rate is a function of the type of disease and the time between recognition and treatment. Case fatality varies widely depending on the type of disease, with strangulating lesions having the highest rate.

Risk factors for colic

Risk factors for colic have been examined in several studies. A risk factor is not necessarily a cause, but indicates that there is an increased risk of colic when a horse is exposed to it. Specific diseases are associated with signalment or other factors. As an example, the foal has a higher risk of

Table 1.1 Type and frequency of colic signs observed in horses with colic

Sign	Frequency (%)
Rolling	44
Continuous or intermittent pawing	43
Lying down for excessive periods of time	29
Lying down repeatedly	21
Turning head toward flank	14
Repeatedly curling the upper lip	13
Backing into corner, uncomfortable	10
Kicking at abdomen	7
Standing in a stretched position	4
Frequent positioning as if to urinate	3
Lack of defecation greater than 24 hours	1

Other signs that can indicate colic include lack of appetite, strange or depressed behaviour, sweating and diarrhoea.
Adapted from Tinker *et al*, (1997).

meconium impaction. Similarly, standard bred horses, Tennessee Walking horses, American Saddlebreds and Warmblood horses are all prone to abnormal enlargement of the inguinal rings, thus predisposing them to inguinal hernia. Tennant and co-workers (1972) noted that ponies were at higher risk for small colon obstruction. Other reported risks (though not proven in all cases) include abdominal abscesses in mares, lipomas in horses 12 years of age and older, enteroliths in California and Florida, and ileal impaction in the south-eastern United States (White, 1990).

Several diseases are associated with specific events or factors. Colic owing to adhesions is most likely to be seen in horses that have had previous abdominal surgery (Cohen *et al.*, 1995). Horses with large colon impactions frequently have a history of an acute increase in stall time, reduced exercise and concurrent medical treatment (Dabareiner and White, 1995). Impactions are also associated with reduced water intake and with the feeding of coarse roughage to horses with poor teeth. Caecal impactions are anecdotally related to treatment with phenylbutazone or in a hospital, and dorsal colitis is associated with phenylbutazone administration. Inguinal hernias occur most frequently either during or immediately after breeding.

When examining risks in the normal population, where idiopathic colic is most common, there appears to no increased risk for sex. Arabian horses are reported to be at higher risk than other breeds, and horses aged 2–10 years have a higher risk of colic than young horses (foals, weanlings and yearlings) or those over 10 years of age (Cohen *et al.*, 1995; Reeves *et al.*, 1989; Tinker *et al*, 1997). Though studies have evaluated risks in slightly different ways, several events appear to increase the risk of colic, including pregnancy, the period of lactation, change in diet, recent change in activity, transport, fever, and vaccination (Cohen *et al.*, 1995; Tinker *et al*, 1997). The risk was found to increase as the amount of grain fed increased, compared to horses not fed grain – those horses fed 2.5 kg/day or more had an increased risk of colic. Horses fed pelleted feeds and commercially mixed sweet feeds also had an increased risk of colic when compared to horses fed no concentrates (Tinker *et al*, 1997). Horses with a previous history of colic were more likely to have colic than horses with no such history (Cohen *et al.*, 1995; Tinker *et al*, 1997).

Classification of colic

Colic is frequently classified by the type of disease observed or by the altered physiological processes that take place during the colic episode. Many of the severe diseases that cause colic can be identified at surgery or necropsy, but the mild cases are often difficult to classify. Many mild episodes are frequently blamed on intestinal spasm (spasmodic colic) or ileus (functional obstruction). Classification of diseases causing colic and examples of each classification are given in Table 1.2.

Based on cause, colic cases can be described as one of seven basic types owing to the following:

1. Diet
2. Anatomical predisposition

Table 1.2 Classification of diseases causing colic, with examples for each classification

Classification	Type of disease	Possible cause
Ileus	Spasm	Unknown
	Intraluminal obstruction	
	impaction	coarse feed
	flatulence	excess fermentation
	occluding mass	foreign bodies
	Paralytic ileus	
	stasis	electrolyte imbalance
	increased tone	sympathomimetic response
	Displacement/strangulation	
	inguinal hernia	anatomic predisposition
	large colon volvulus	abnormal motility
Inflammation	Enteritis	
	thrombotic colic	verminous arteritis
	colitis	Salmonella sp.
	abscess	*Streptococcus equi*
	toxins	cantharidin
Ulcer	Gastric ulcers (squamous)	unknown
	Gastric ulcers (glandular)	NSAIDs
	Intestinal ulcers	NSAIDs
	Dorsal colitis	NSAIDs
False colic	Pregnancy	uterine contractions
	Rhabdomyolitis	exertional myositis
	Liver disease	toxic plants
	Renal/bladder	bladder stone
	Pleuritis	pneumonia
	Psychogenic	vice

3. Alterations in motility
4. Infection
5. Parasites
6. Ulceration
7. Alternate organs or systems.

The majority of colic cases observed are due to intestinal disease, and 80–90 per cent of these are classified as a form of ileus, as there is no known cause, or descriptive terms such as spasmodic or gas colic are applied. An understanding of the types of colic is helpful in making the diagnosis, and is useful for investigating colic in individual horses or groups of horses.

Classification of colic based on the segment of intestine involved and the type of obstruction reveals the case fatality of specific diseases. When examining the records from 14 university hospitals, the large colon (28.6 per cent) and small intestine (19.1 per cent) were the most commonly affected bowel segments. Case fatality was highest for the rectum (82.1 per cent), followed by the stomach (77.7 per cent), primarily due to rectal tears and gastric rupture. Diseases of the small intestine, caecum and large and small colons had case fatality rates of 67.3 per cent, 55.6 per cent, 40.5 per cent and 34.7 per cent respectively, reflecting the relative rate of strangulating diseases seen in each respective segment (White, 1990).

Causes of colic

There are numerous causes of colic, though the causes of most colic episodes are unknown.

Parasites have been shown to cause colic, and parasite control programmes have reduced its incidence, specifically implicating small strongyle infection as a cause (Uhlinger, 1990). Small strongyle migration can cause inflammation, and it has been speculated that it might cause alterations in motility. Large strongyles cause alterations in the cranial mesenteric vasculature, and can cause thromboembolic colic (White, 1981). Tapeworm infection has been associated with caecal and ileocaecal problems, and has been shown to be a risk factor (Proudman and Edwards, 1993).

Ingestion of foreign materials can cause colic. Sand can collect in the colon and eventually cause obstruction, and ingestion of foreign bodies such as nails, wire or stones with sharp edges can initiate enterolith formation. Colon pH must be increased to allow enterolith formation, but the relationship of pH and mineral concentrations needed to form enteroliths is not understood. Other foreign materials that are recognized causes of intestinal obstruction include rubber fencing (Boles and Kohn, 1977), nylon materials (such as carpet, halter straps), hair (tricholiths) and seeds.

Trauma can result in abdominal injuries, which may result in bowel entrapment or displacement. Mesenteric rents have been associated with abdominal trauma and difficulties during foaling. These rents do not become evident until the intestine becomes incarcerated, and often strangulated, months later. Haematomas of the bowel wall are rare, but are seen in the small intestine and the small colon.

Congenital problems can be responsible for colic, and include obstruction due to volvulus or incarceration from a mesodiverticular band or ileus due to aganglionosis in paint foals from an inherited lethal white gene (White, 1990). Atresia coli, inguinal hernia, diaphragmatic hernia and mesenteric defects are other congenital defects that can lead to intestinal obstruction and colic.

Enteritis due to inflammation of the mucosa or the intestinal wall can cause colic, but the colic is often short-lived, and is not the predominant sign for these problems. Salmonella can cause colic in its early stages and, similarly, equine erhliciosis (Potomac Horse Fever) may have colic as one of its signs. Idiopathic peritonitis can also cause colic. Post-operative peritonitis can cause colic, or may be associated with ileus or obstruction, which is the primary cause of colic. The common signs for most of these inflammatory diseases include fever, depression and diarrhoea.

Infection of the abdominal cavity is usually caused by injured intestine, although haematogenous infection is possible. Prior surgery can also be a source of infection, due to contamination at surgery, leakage from an anastomotic site or degeneration of bowel after surgery. Peritonitis causes colic, but this is often intermittent and due to irritation of the serosa. Infection of the mesenteric lymphatics can cause mesenteric abscesses due to *Streptococcus equi* and Rodococcus spp. Subsequent adhesions of the intestines cause obstruction and subsequent colic.

Toxins are rare, but can result in colic. Cantharidin, from Blister beetles, can cause severe enteritis with colic. Monensin™, a feed additive for cattle and poultry feeds, can also cause colic if fed to horses. Amitraz™, an arachnidcide, is an alpha agonist which causes cessation of colon motility. Grass sickness, though a generalized disease, has gut stasis and colic as one of its signs.

Gastrointestinal ulcers are a cause of colic (Murray, 1992), and foals with gastric ulcers have colic as one of the possible signs. These foals generally have ulceration of the squamous portion of the mucosa, though glandular ulcers do occur and older foals (4–6 months) can have duodenal ulcers, which cause abnormal gastric emptying. Ulcers in adult horses do not cause colic as frequently as in foals, and the ulcers are generally seen in the squamous portion of the stomach. Signs of ulcers are predominantly poor appetite, poor condition or poor performance; however, severe ulcers have been responsible for severe colic, with signs indicating the need for surgery.

Gastric and intestinal ulcers may be seen following chronic administration of non-steroidal anti-inflammatory drugs (NSAIDs). These ulcers are found in the glandular mucosa, and are related to suppression of prostaglandin E_2. Horses with phenylbutazone toxicosis can have colic as one of the signs, and this normally starts mildly and becomes chronic.

Ileus is a general term that refers to intestinal obstruction. This can be physical obstruction, but the term will be used here to indicate abnormal motility, which can include paralytic ileus, ileus caused by distension, or malposition of the intestine from abnormal motility. Incarcerations, volvulus and intestinal displacement are included in this group.

The causes of intestinal spasm, atony, impaction or alterations in intestinal position are not known. Suspected causes include systemic electrolyte imbalances (specifically hypocalcaemia), parasite infections, systemic dehydration, abnormal intestinal bacterial growth or changes in the intestinal pH. It is likely that diseases such as small intestinal volvulus have more than one predisposing cause – as an example, the length of mesentery and abnormal movement of the intestine are both generally necessary for a volvulus to occur. Presently, all mechanisms are speculative because of a lack of understanding about the patho-physiology of intestinal motility and possible alterations in intestinal physiology.

Alterations in both calcium and potassium serum levels have been associated with colic and implicated as causes of ileus. Reduced serum calcium can cause ileus, and is frequently observed in horses with colon displacements and other acute episodes of colic. The reason for the lowered serum calcium is unknown, and it is not known if the lowered calcium precedes the colic episode or is a result of the intestinal problem. Low serum potassium does not directly cause colic as low calcium does, but administration of potassium during hypokalemia can improve intestinal motility. Magnesium is also known to cause alterations in motility, and this problem is usually seen in horses with a form of grass tetany where both magnesium and calcium are low, or in horses who have been off feed for long periods.

The caecum and colon are part of a fermentation system that digests cellulose, with the subsequent formation of volatile fatty acids. Feeding routines incorporating twice-daily feeding cause alterations in systemic hydration due to the secretion of water into the colon to balance the osmotic effect of the rapidly forming fatty acids (Clarke and Argenzio, 1990). A rapid drop in pH and filling of the colon may lead to stasis or, subsequently, the fatty acid and water absorption from the colon lumen may cause a relative dehydration of ingesta. These events are speculated to cause abnormal motility, but there is no proof that they influence either motility or the risk of colic. Impaction of the large colon is one of the most common diseases causing colic, though the cause remains a mystery. Risk factors such as increased grain intake and changes in activity or diet may be causes of colic, or may be related to these alterations in gut function, which can lead to colic.

False colic

False colic is the term used to describe signs similar to those in intestinal tract colic but caused by another organ system. False colic may be a sign of rhabdomyolysis, which can cause changes in heart rate, anxiety and body movements such as pawing and turning the head toward the body. Renal and bladder diseases can cause colic but are rare in horses, although ruptured bladder may occur in foals. Pleuritis, myocardial infarction and liver and uterine disease can all cause colic that is indistinguishable from an acute abdomen (White, 1990). The signs of colic can be behavioural and, though rare, horses have habitually shown colic for different stimuli – eating has been reported (Murray and Crowell Davis, 1985).

References

Boles, C. L. and Kohn, C. W. (1977). Fibrous foreign body impaction colic in young horses. *J. Am. Vet. Med. Assoc.*, **171**, 193–5.

Clarke, L. L. R. M. and Argenzio, R. A. (1990). Feeding and digestive problems in horses physiologic responses to a concentrated meal. *Vet. Clin. N. Am. Equine Pract.*, **6**, 433–49.

Cohen, N. D., Matejka, P. L., Honnas, C. M. and Hooper, R. N. (1995). Case–control study of the association between various management factors and development of colic in horses. Texas Equine Colic Study Group. *J. Am. Vet. Med. Assoc.*, **206**, 667–73.

Dabareiner, D. M. and White, N. A. (1995). Large colon impaction in horses: 147 cases (1985–1991). *J. Am. Vet. Med. Assoc.*, **206**, 679–85.

Murray, M. J. (1992). Gastric ulceration in horses: 91 cases (1987–1990). *J. Am. Vet. Med. Assoc.*, **201**, 117–20.

Murray, M. J. and Crowell Davis, S. L. (1985). Psychogenic colic in a horse. *J. Am. Vet. Med. Assoc.*, **186**, 381–3.

Proudman, C. J. and Edwards, G. B. (1993). Are tapeworms associated with equine colic? A case–control study. *Equine Vet. J.*, **25**, 224–6.

Reeves, M. J., Gay, J. M., Hilbert, B. J. and Morris, R. S. (1989). Association of age, sex and breed factors in acute equine colic: a retrospective study of 320 cases admitted to a veterinary teaching hospital in the USA. *Prev. Vet. Med.*, **7**, 149–60.

Rollins, J. B. and Clement, T. H. (1979). Observations on incidence of equine colic in a private practice. *Equine Pract.*, **1**, 39–42.

Tennant, B., Wheat, J. D. and Meagher, D. M. (1972). Observations on the causes and incidence of acute intestinal obstruction in the horse. *Proceedings 18th Annual Convention of the AAEP*, pp. 251–258.

Tinker, M. K., Lessard, P., Thatcher, C. D. *et al* (1997). Prospective study of equine colic incidence and mortality. *Equine Vet. J.*, **29(6)**, 449.

Uhlinger, C. (1990). Effects of three anthelmintic schedules on the incidence of colic in horses. *Equine Vet. J.*, **22(4)**, 251–4.

Uhlinger, C. (1992). Investigations into the incidence of field colic. *Equine Vet. J.*, **13**, 11–18.

White, N. A. (1981). Intestinal infarction associated with mesenteric vascular thrombotic disease in the horse. *J. Am. Vet. Med. Assoc.*, **178**, 259–62.

White, N. A. (1990). Epidemiology and etiology of colic. In *The Equine Acute Abdomen* (N. A. White, ed.), pp. 50–64. Lea and Febiger.

2

Examination of the horse

Introduction

Acute abdominal pain is a relatively frequent occurrence and the majority of cases, probably greater than 90 per cent, respond readily to medical therapy. The primary aim of the initial examination is to distinguish horses with a mild or uncomplicated disease process from those with a potentially life-threatening disorder requiring further monitoring, surgery or intensive care. The earlier these serious disorders are recognized and specific therapy instituted, the better is the prognosis for recovery.

Whether a diagnosis can be made at the initial examination or requires the procedure to be repeated on one or more occasions will depend on the cause of the colic and the length of time it has been in existence. It is important that the results are carefully documented so that findings recorded at successive examinations can be compared and important trends in the course of the illness recognized.

History

The most important factor of the history is the time that has elapsed since the onset of colic. This may be known precisely, but can often only be estimated – for example, in the case of horses found in colic at the owner's first inspection of the day, having last been seen normal the previous evening. It is essential that a reasonably accurate assessment of the likely duration be made in order that the significance of the clinical findings can be evaluated.

The remainder of the history should include the general history relating to husbandry and management, the recent history and management, and more specific details related to the present colic episode.

The general history may not help to identify the specific cause of the episode of colic under investigation, but information such as inadequate anthelmintic treatment may be important. A history of previous illness may be significant; for example, in a horse with chronic intermittent colic, an episode of strangles several weeks earlier may suggest a mesenteric abscess. A higher incidence of sand colic or enterolithiasis may be known to be associated with particular areas of the country. Recent changes in housing or bedding materials or qualitative or quantitative changes in feed may be directly involved. For example, horses brought in from pasture and bedded on straw may eat the bedding in preference to hay, and develop large colon impaction as a consequence.

Previous treatments may lead to gastrointestinal disease. As examples, anthelmintic treatment of foals which have a heavy ascarid burden can lead to small intestine obstruction with dead worms, while other medications such as non-steroidal anti-inflammatory drugs (NSAIDs) have the potential for toxicity.

Questions relating to the present colic episode should specifically address the following points:

1. How severe has the pain been, and has it altered during the time the horse has been observed?
2. When did the horse last defecate, and what was the character of the faeces?
3. Has the horse shown specific behaviour, such as playing with water or adopting abnormal postures?
4. Could the horse have gained access to too much highly fermentable food?
5. Is there any association with change of exercise routine, parturition or mating?

Physical examination

Manifestations of pain

Whilst the history is being taken, the horse may be inspected in its stall and the nature and degree of colicky signs currently being shown noted. In response to mild gastrointestinal pain, the horse may occasionally paw the ground, turn its head to its flank, stretch out or lie down for longer than normal. When moderate pain is present, the horse may kick at its abdomen, repeatedly crouch as if about to lie down, and lie down and roll. If the pain is severe, sweating, dropping to the ground, violent rolling, groaning and continuous movement are the signs usually displayed. In general, the more severe the disease, the greater the pain, but all diseases can show a wide spectrum of signs.

Skin abrasions about the eyes and over the tuber coxae are indicative of rolling and other violent behaviour prompted by severe pain. Marks on the wall of the box caused by the horse kicking and excessive disturbance of the bedding are further evidence of severe pain consistent with a severe obstruction. Horses with an obstruction or strangulation that has arisen only within the past 4–5 hours or so exhibit signs of severe pain, whereas those in which the problem is of much longer duration and where the segment of gut has undergone advanced necrosis show few signs of overt pain. In these cases, although apparently calm, horses have signs of severe depression – for example, standing with the head held low and taking no interest in the surroundings. This 'stage of indolence' is associated with severe endotoxaemia. Such an evaluation of the circumstantial evidence and presenting signs at the time of examination allows a reasonably accurate assessment of the duration of the problem when the time of onset is not known. Other signs to note are evidence of abdominal distension, and umbilical or unilateral scrotal enlargement.

After taking the history and observing the horse, the veterinarian should now proceed to a systematic physical examination.

Assessment of shock

Pulse

The heart rate and character of the pulse are important criteria in assessing the colic patient. In general, pain and the activity as a consequence of pain have only a relatively minor effect on heart rate, which is influenced much more by haemoconcentration and diminished venous return and by the cardiovascular response to endotoxaemia. There is a close relationship between the pulse rate and the nature and duration of the colic. Whereas horses with pelvic flexure impaction show little or no elevation, even when the obstruction has been present for 48 hours, those with ileal impaction have a progressive rise in pulse rate as hypovolaemia develops in response to the sequestration of fluid in the small intestine and stomach. Infarctive disease is usually accompanied by a non-fluctuating elevation in heart rate, which increases progressively as endotoxic shock develops. How rapidly this increase occurs depends to a significant degree on the amount of distension and length of the compromised intestine.

Generally, the pulse rate is an indicator of the severity of the disease and its effect on the cardiovascular system. Rates greater than 80 bpm should be considered the result of a severe lesion or disease, which is producing severe cardiovascular compromise and is therefore more likely to be fatal. The character of the pulse should also be evaluated. A weak pulse is usually associated with shock and lowered vascular volume. Acute electrolyte imbalance can result in an irregular pulse.

Respiration

Horses with moderate to severe abdominal pain will usually have a respiratory rate of above 30 per minute in an apparent attempt to reduce movement of the diaphragm and chest. Pressure on the diaphragm by a grossly distended large colon will similarly elevate the respiratory rate, as will acidosis or herniation of intestine into the pleural space. Elevation of the respiratory rate accompanied by cyanosis due to compression of the vena cava or pulmonary damage from endotoxin or hypovolaemia is evidence of a life-threatening disease.

Mucous membranes

The character of the mucous membranes is important in determining the hydration of the horse. The gingiva (provided they are not pigmented) provide the best surface for assessment because the conjunctivae are often congested due to trauma. The oral mucous membranes are normally pale pink, but variation in this colour results from dehydration, depending on the cause. Simple dehydration causes slight blanching of the mucosae, but with venous congestion or endotoxin release they become red to brick red and eventually cyanotic. Terminally, due to dramatically reduced perfusion and hypoxia, the membranes are a pale blue-grey colour.

Tissue perfusion and cardiovascular performance can be assessed by evaluating the capillary refill time. After pressure has been applied to the gingiva above the incisor teeth, the time normally taken for the blanched area to return to its original colour is 1–2 seconds. In the dehydrated horse this is lengthened to 3–4 seconds, and when severe dehydration is present this extends to 5–6 seconds.

Assessment of intestinal movement

Auscultation

The abdomen should be thoroughly auscultated, the best sites being along the caudal edge of the rib cage from paralumbar fossa to ventral abdomen on both right and left sides. In the normal horse there are two types of large intestinal sounds: short, mixing sounds, which occur two to four times per minute; and long, propulsive (toilet flush) sounds, which occur once every two to four minutes but which increase in frequency and magnitude after the horse eats. In almost all cases of abdominal pain, the propulsive sounds are decreased. The obvious exception is spasmodic colic, in which increased sounds may be very obvious, allowing the case to be classified as mild medical and given an excellent prognosis. Increased sounds may also be heard following resolution of ileus in tympanic or simple colic cases. The sounds may be reduced or even absent for 20–60 minutes or more after the administration of drugs such as xylazine, detomidine and butorphanol.

Colonic impactions have reduced intestinal sounds, which usually coincide with bouts of abdominal pain. In cases of severe intestinal disease, such as strangulations, all sounds are absent within a few hours of the obstruction occurring. Gas/fluid interface sounds caused by movement of the horse should not be mistaken for propulsive sounds. Evidence of increased intraluminal fluid may be detected in colitis cases just prior to the onset of diarrhoea. Excessive caecal or colonic gas may be detected in primary flatulent colic or tympany secondary to displacements. Unlike in ruminants, abdominal percussion and/or ballotment are rarely helpful, but palpation of the abdominal wall is important in identifying 'boarding' or 'splinting' in response to generalized peritonitis due to rupture of the stomach or intestine.

Transit

Measurement of intestinal transit time is not considered a diagnostic procedure in horses with colic, but has been used as an experimental tool to evaluate the efficacy of drugs to restore propulsive activity.

Mineral oil, which will normally pass from stomach to rectum in 12–18 hours, is administered by some veterinarians as a fluid marker to eliminate the possibility of a complete obstruction. However, its use should, in the author's opinion, be restricted to diagnosed cases of primary large colon impaction. It should never be given to a horse suspected of having any form of strangulation obstruction or to a horse with severe pain where the diagnosis cannot be made. In these cases, it can complicate the problem. In horses with small intestinal obstruction, mineral oil or other laxative can add to the gastric dilatation and increase the risk of rupture.

Diagnostic aids

Gastric reflux

Nasogastric intubation should be carried out routinely in all colic cases. In addition to being of diagnostic value, decompression of the stomach produces immediate alleviation of pain and reduces the risk of rupture. Gastric tympany may be released spontaneously following intubation, but to remove gastric fluid it is usually necessary to create a siphon by adding a small volume of water to the tube then lowering it below the level of the stomach (Fig. 2.1). Alternatively, suction may be applied to the tube or a stomach pump used in reverse. If no fluid is refluxed, the

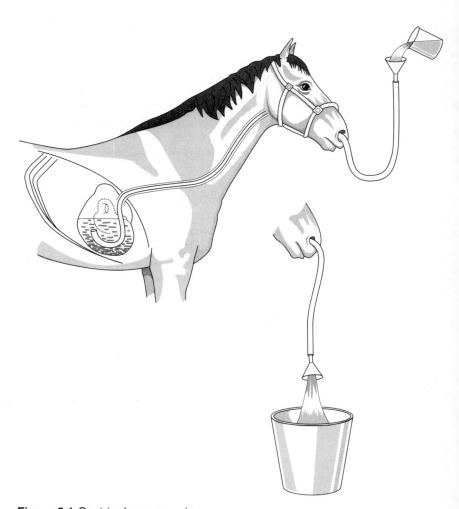

Figure 2.1 Gastric decompression.

tube should be repositioned by advancing or withdrawing it several inches and the siphon procedure repeated. At least five attempts should be made, particularly if distended small intestine is palpable on rectal examination. Gastric reflux of more than 2 l is considered to be significant, and usually indicates a primary disorder located in the stomach or small intestine. However, in some large colon displacements the duodenum is compressed, preventing normal gastric emptying. Grass sickness, anterior enteritis, ileus and peritonitis can also cause gastric distension. Normal gastric fluid has a pH of 3–6, but following intestinal obstruction it changes to 6–8 due to the buffering effect of fluid from the small intestine.

Rectal examination

Rectal examination is the single most important part of the clinical examination of the horse with colic, and should always be performed unless the animal is too small or too violent. In each case the rectal examination must be approached with respect to both its value and the risks involved.

While rectal examination is of considerable value in the diagnosis of benign problems such as primary impaction and tympany of the large intestine and hyperactivity of intestine in spasmodic colic, it is of greater importance in recognizing those cases that require surgical intervention. Many of the cases can be diagnosed by rectal palpation before the animal becomes very ill or peritoneal fluid changes become apparent. The early diagnosis and referral of these cases significantly improves the prognosis and reduces the occurrence of post-operative complications.

Adequate restraint is essential to prevent damage to the horse or examiner. When rectal examination is performed in a stable or barn, restraint may comprise the use of a twitch, chemical restraint such as xylazine or raising a foreleg. If the veterinarian uses the left hand for rectal examination, the horse should be positioned with its left flank against the wall and the head restrained on the right side. Stocks provide a safeguard against being kicked, but the examiner must always be wary of the horse suddenly attempting to go down, putting the examiner's arm and horse's rectum at risk of injury.

Adequate lubrication of the rectal sleeve with methyl cellulose, slow introduction of the hand and arm into the rectum, and being prepared to withdraw them if confronted with a strong peristaltic wave will minimize the risk of damage to the rectum. Care should be taken to ensure no tail hairs are carried into the rectum, and all faeces within reach must be removed prior to any attempt to palpate structures. Once the arm has been introduced to its full length, it is advisable to hold it still for 30 seconds, during which time the colon usually relaxes. In particularly difficult cases, injecting 60 ml of xylocaine into the rectum or applying xylocaine gel to the rectal sleeve may be helpful. The abdominal and pelvic contents should be palpated by running the hand along the surfaces, rather than by grasping structures through the rectal wall. At the end of any examination, the hand should be checked for any evidence of blood. If there is any concern that a rectal tear has occurred, greater sensitivity is achieved by wearing a plastic sleeve with the fingers cut off and a surgical glove placed over the hand.

A systematic examination should always be performed, bearing in mind that it is limited to the caudal 40 per cent of the abdomen even in small horses and ponies. In basic terms, the questions to be answered are as follows:

1. Is the position of the viscera normal?
2. Is there distension of intestine?
3. If distension is present:
    Is it due to ingesta, fluid or gas?
    Is it distension of the caecum, colon or small intestine?
4. Are there any other findings of note, e.g. abnormal motility, presence of sand, abnormal peritoneal surfaces or blood in the faeces?

The normal structures palpable (Fig. 2.2a and b) include, in the left dorsal quadrant, the spleen, the caudal pole of the left kidney and, linking the two, the nephrosplenic ligament. Moving to the right and extending forwards below the spine, the root of the mesentery can be palpated, although in large horses this may be difficult. Specific arterial identification may be impossible, and it is frequently easier to identify the caecocolic artery at the base of the caecum than to palpate the cranial mesenteric artery. In the right dorsal quadrant, the base of the caecum is identified. Normally the caecum is not full, and the caudal and medial bands running from the dorsal to the ventral aspects are fairly relaxed and allow the fingers to be hooked around one or other of them and traction applied to the caecum. Moving ventral to the pelvic brim, the pelvic flexure of the large colon containing soft ingesta can usually be detected and, extending cranially from it, the large diameter left ventral colon with its clearly recognized longitudinal bands, and the narrow, smooth left dorsal colon. The normal small intestine is usually not palpable unless it happens to contract when touched, but the small colon is easily recognized by the formed faecal balls it contains. The inguinal canals can be felt in the stallion to either side of the pelvic opening at the pubic brim. The bladder, when distended, can limit palpation of organs cranial to it. Stimulating the horse to urinate by placing it in a clean box, or evacuating the bladder by catheterization, will overcome this problem.

Although specific diagnoses can be made on the basis of rectal findings, more often the examiner can discern only distension of a specific segment of bowel, or a particular position that identifies an obstruction.

Diseases of the stomach are rarely identifiable on rectal examination. The spleen may give the impression of being pushed caudally by gastric distension, but splenic enlargement will mimic this finding. Rarely, a massively impacted stomach may be palpable.

Small intestine

Obstruction or adynamic ileus of the small intestine produces distension recognizable by one or more loops containing gas and fluid. The number of palpable loops depends on the nature, duration and location of the lesion. In the early stages of obstruction, careful, patient palpation over several minutes may be necessary before a distended loop is recognized. As the intestine continues to distend, it folds onto itself, forming

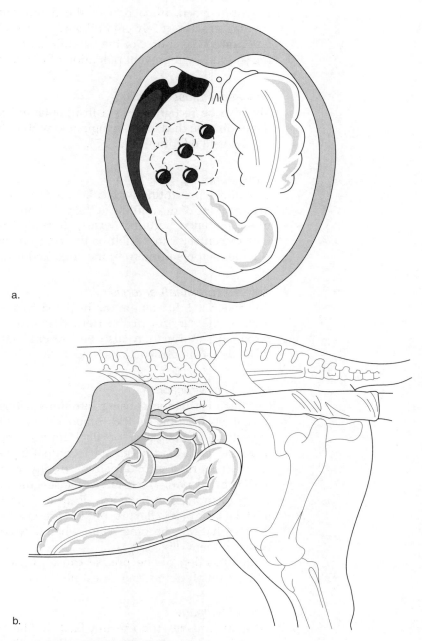

Figure 2.2 a. Normal findings
b. Normal findings.

accordion-like loops positioned vertically or horizontally and occupying any quadrant of the abdomen. The cause of the obstruction is identified only infrequently (Fig. 2.3a and b).

Ileal impaction
If within reach, impaction of the ileum can be recognized as a firm tubular structure 12–16 cm in diameter medial to the base of the caecum. Later on in the course of the condition, distension of much, if not all, of the jejunum will prevent palpation of the ileum (Fig. 2.4).

Ileocaecal intussusception
This can be recognized as a firm, enlarged tubular or coiled structure, depending on the length invaginated within the base of the caecum in the right dorsal quadrant (Fig. 2.5).

Inguinal hernia
In stallions presenting with colic, palpation of the internal inguinal rings to either side of the midline at the pubic rim should always be performed. In strangulated inguinal hernia, distended painful small intestine and taut mesentery can be felt at the ring on the same side as the scrotal enlargement resulting from the engorged testis.

Anterior (proximal) enteritis
The distended duodenum can be palpated as a tubular structure over the base of the caecum in the right dorsal quadrant. Some distension of proximal jejunum may also be present, but the gut is not so tightly distended as in obstructions (Fig. 2.6).

Chronic obstruction
Chronic obstruction causing intermittent bouts of colic may be due to partial obstruction of the lumen of the small intestine by muscular hypertrophy, neoplasia or ileal intussusception. As a result of the increased workload necessary to propel ingesta through the constricted segment, marked secondary hypertrophy occurs in the intestine proximal to the obstruction. The result is that several metres dilate to a diameter of 10 cm or more, and have a wall up to 1 cm thick. A single loop can be mistaken for pelvic flexure, but the presence of other identical loops, and the fact that they become 'solid' when they contract, helps to distinguish between them (Fig. 2.7).

Identification of the precise cause of the obstruction is more likely when it involves the large intestine.

Caecal tympany
Tympany pushes the caecum back to the pelvic inlet, and the tense ventral taenia can be felt running diagonally from the right dorsal to the left ventral quadrant. The distension can fill all quadrants (Fig. 2.8).

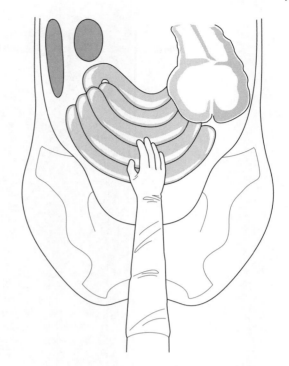

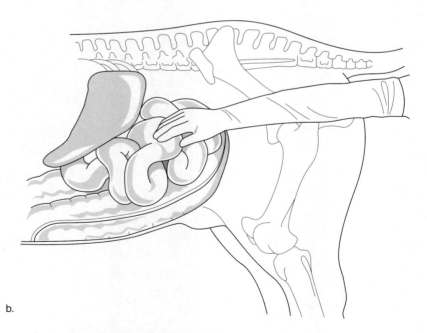

Figure 2.3 a. Small intestine obstruction
b. Small intestine distension.

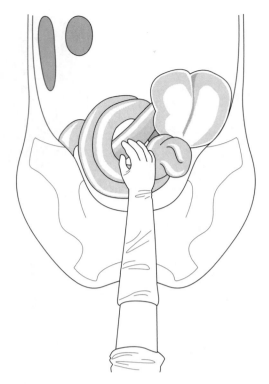

Figure 2.4 Ileal impaction.

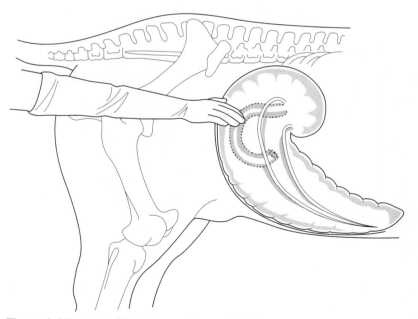

Figure 2.5 Ileocaecal intussusception.

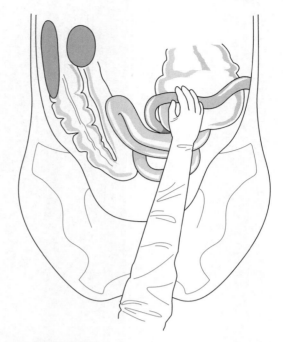

Figure 2.6 Proximal enteritis.

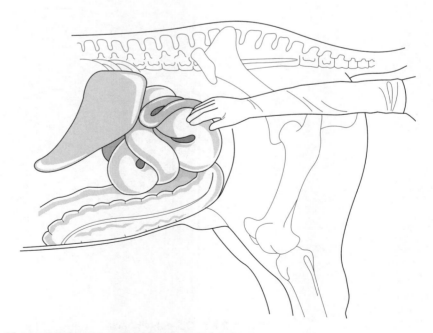

Figure 2.7 Chronic small intestine obstruction.

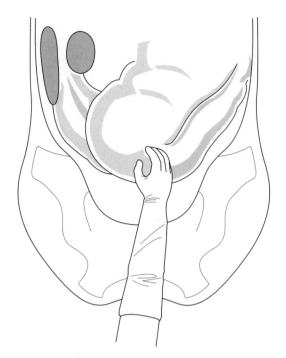

a.

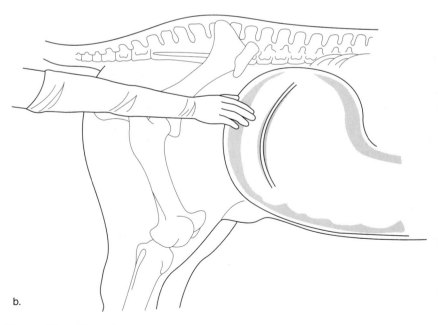

b.

Figure 2.8 a. Caecal tympany
b. Caecal tympany.

Caecal impaction

Caecal impaction presents as a viscus filled with hard digesta and with a distinct ventral band. A hand can be passed to the right of, but not dorsal to, the viscus. Typically, the caecal base fills before the body and little or no gaseous distension is evident. In some cases, the distension is massive and the ingest has a semi-fluid character. In these cases rupture is often imminent.

Caeco-caecal intussusception

The firm, oedematous, invaginated body portion of the caecum can sometimes be palpated within the base (Fig. 2.9).

Large colon

Large colon impaction is characterized by an enlarged, firm, evenly-filled viscus, which is often located on the pelvic floor or alternatively just below the pelvis to the left or right (Fig. 2. 10).

In left dorsal displacement (nephrosplenic entrapment), varying lengths of left colon are draped over the nephrosplenic ligament. If the displaced portion is large, the bands hang down in a diagonal direction and the pelvic flexure cannot be palpated (Fig. 2.11a). An impaction is often palpable in the left dorsal colon just caudal to the nephrosplenic ligament (Fig. 2.11b). Considerable tympany of the left ventral portion may obscure the spleen. If only a short length of colon lies caudal to the spleen, the impacted pelvic flexure is easily recognized. In cases of incomplete entrapment, the spleen deviates away from the left

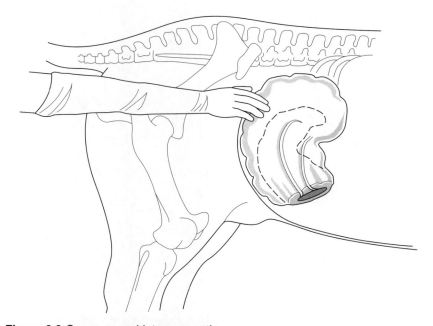

Figure 2.9 Caeco-caecal intussusception.

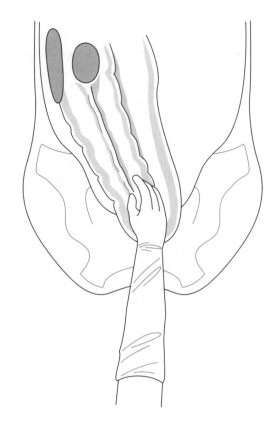

a.

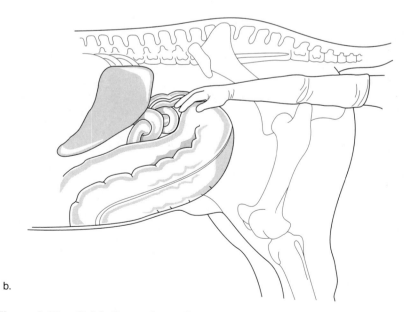

b.

Figure 2.10 a. Pelvic flexure impaction
b. Large colon impaction.

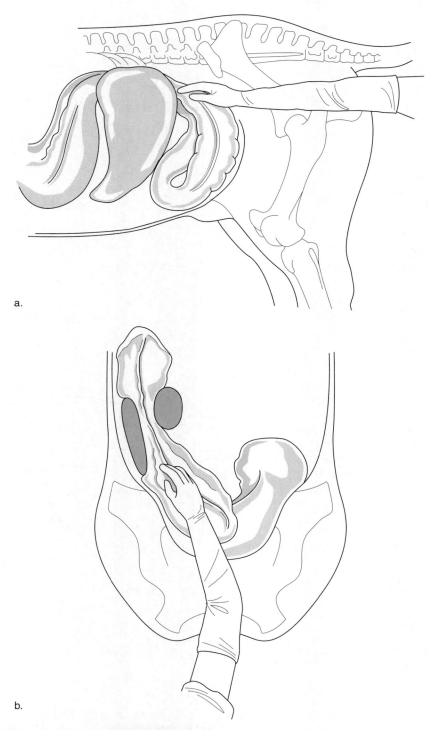

a.

b.

Figure 2.11 a. Left dorsal displacement
b. Left dorsal displacement.

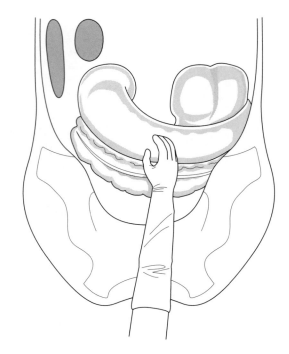

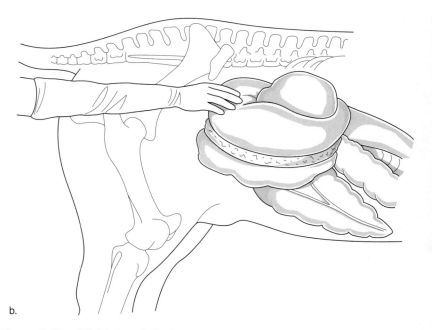

Figure 2.12 a. Right dorsal displacement
b. Right dorsal displacement.

abdominal wall. In some cases the colon can be followed into the nephrosplenic space.

During right dorsal displacement, the slight to moderately distended large colon lies horizontally in front of the pelvic canal, caudal to the tympanitic caecum. The caecum is positioned away from the right abdominal wall. The mesocolon, containing fat and large vessels, can be recognized and traced to the right, where it can be felt passing between the caecum and the abdominal wall. Oedema of the mesocolon, when present, indicates a degree of torsion (Fig. 2.12).

Severe large colon torsion produces such great distension it is often impossible to explore beyond the pelvic inlet. The characteristic features are a horizontal colon with palpable thickening of its wall and mesocolon due to oedema. Occasionally it can be in a vertical position (Fig. 2.13).

Caecal decompression

Caecal trocharization can be performed easily and safely, requiring no special instrumentation. When performed properly, the benefits (in the form of relief of the severe pain and restoration of normal gastrointestinal function) far outweigh the risks in patients with extreme tympany.

Technique
1. The area over the right paralumbar region in which the resonant ping is most consistently detected is clipped and aseptically prepared prior

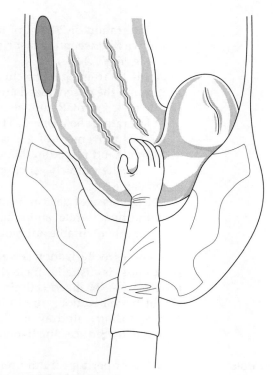

Figure 2.13 Large colon volvulus.

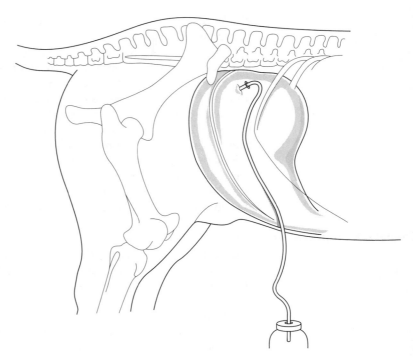

Figure 2.14 Caecal decompression.

to infiltration of 2–3 ml of local anaesthetic into the skin and muscle midway between the last rib and the ventral prominence of the tuber coxae (Fig. 2.14).

2. A 14- to 16-gauge 12.5 cm (5 in) intravenous catheter is introduced through the desensitized area perpendicular to the skin and advanced into the caecum. Removal of the stylet at this stage will reduce the risk of lacerating the caecum. The catheter is left in place in the caecum as long as movement of gas is detected. Gentle pressure on the caecum from a hand placed in the rectum will assist in the escape of gas (Fig. 2.15). Alternatively, suction can be applied if such equipment is available.

3. Once release of gas can no longer be detected, the catheter is quickly withdrawn while simultaneously injecting 5 ml of gentamycin or some other suitable antibiotic.

A single trocharization is well tolerated by the animal. Although a mild peritonitis is usually incited, it does not commonly cause clinical problems. A localized cellulitis may occur in the abdominal wall at the site of trocharization, due to introduction of enteric organisms into the tissues during withdrawal of the catheter. The antibiotic injected at the time greatly reduces the likelihood of this complication.

Abdominocentesis

Analysis of peritoneal fluid reflects the changes that occur in tissues and organs within the abdominal cavity and on the peritoneal surface. In colic

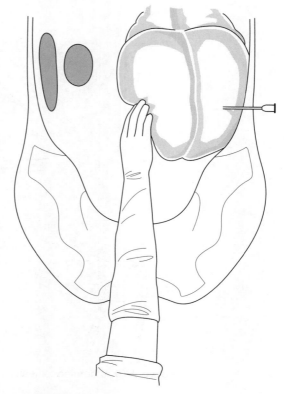

Figure 2.15 Caecal decompression.

cases, it assists in determining the type of disease and the severity of the lesion.

Technique

Abdominocentesis is a safe and simple procedure, which can be performed with a needle or a blunt cannula. The simplest technique is to use a 19-gauge 3.75 cm (1.5 in) needle introduced through a prepared site on the ventral abdominal midline. A dependent point is chosen, and the needle is inserted directly in the midline so that it passes through the linea alba. Entry of the needle into the peritoneal cavity is usually indicated by the flow of varying amounts of fluid, which is collected in a tube with or without EDTA depending on the information required. If no fluid is obtained immediately, slightly withdrawing the needle and/or rotating the hub gently may initiate flow of fluid, as may the introduction of a second needle a few inches from the first, allowing air to enter the abdomen and thus reducing the vacuum. In obese animals, a longer needle may be necessary to penetrate the thick layer of retroperitoneal fat. Contamination of the sample with blood (abdominal wall vessels or spleen) or intestinal contents can complicate interpretation although, if

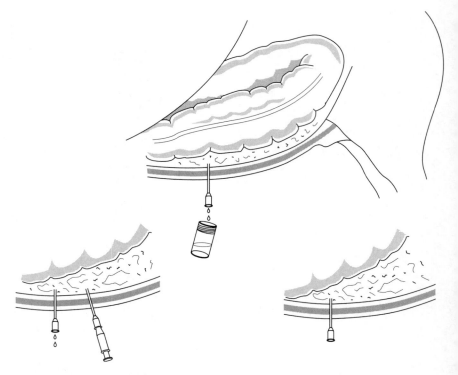

Figure 2.16 Abdominocentesis.

this is recognized at the time of collection, this can be flushed clear with peritoneal fluid by repositioning the needle.

Analysis
The fluid obtained is evaluated by gross visual examination, total protein determination and, if necessary, microscopic examination (Tables 2.1, 2.2, 2.3). Normal fluid is pale yellow and clear. As the fluid changes with specific diseases, it can become more turbid due to increases in protein, RBC and WBC.

Normal peritoneal fluid has < 15 gm/l of protein and no red blood cells. The white cell count is variable, but < 5000 cells/µl is considered normal, the neutrophil : macrophage ratio being 2 : 1. Early in the course of obstructive lesions, the peritoneal fluid remains unchanged. Simple obstruction of intestine results in a slow rise in the protein level without any concurrent rise in blood cells. Strangulation obstruction, however, quickly leads to clearly visible discoloration of the fluid due to leakage of red blood cells within 1–2 hours of the onset of ischaemia. The colour in these early stages varies from pale orange to serosanguinous, depending on the severity of the ischaemia and the length of gut involved, and in some cases the fluid may need to be centrifuged to confirm the presence of red blood cells. As mucosal necrosis occurs, neutrophils increase

Table 2.1 Peritoneal fluid

	Protein	WBC	RBC
Normal	0.7–1.5 g/dl	200–3000/µl neutrophils : monuclear cells 2 : 1	Rarely present
Simple obstruction	Raised	Normal	Normal
Strangulation obstruction	Increased > 2.0 g/dl	Increase as lesion progresses 5×10^3–50×10^3 µl + increase in neutrophils when intestinal necrosis present. WBCs are degenerate and contain intracellular bacteria.	Early increase
Non-strangulating infarction (thrombo-embolic colic)	Raised > 2.0–65 g/dl	Normal to 400 000 µl free and intracellular bacteria	Normal to serosanguinous
Anterior enteritis	Raised 2.0 to 6.5 g/dl	Normal until late stages, when raised	Variable
Post-surgery	Raised	> 5000/µl > 90% neutrophils	$> 20 \times 10^3$
Response to abdominal trauma			
Laparotomy	3.5–6.8 g/dl 1–5 days post-op.	300–450×10^3 µl 1–5 days post-op.	
Laparoscopy	1.4–3.3 g/dl 24 hours post-op.	20–43×10^3 µl 24 hours post-op.	

Table 2.2 Peritoneal fluid cytology

RBC	Crenation is seen commonly
WBC	Karyolisis – indicator of sepsis Karorhexis – end product of nuclear breakdown Toxic change – bluish tinge to vacuoles in cytoplasm
All phagocytosis	Macrophages remove dead WBCs
Free bacteria	

Table 2.3 Peritoneal fluid chemistry

Alkaline phosphatase	isoenzyme increased in small intestine disease
CK	raised above serum levels in ischaemic bowel disease
Creatine	raised above serum levels in foals with bladder rupture
Lactate	raised when bowel degeneration present

progressively as intestinal degeneration progresses. The number of white blood cells can vary from 5000–100 000+; 90–95 per cent are neutrophils, and these undergo degenerative changes due to stimulation by bacteria and toxins. A smear of peritoneal fluid on a slide stained with Wright's stain enables the types and proportion of cells and the presence and extent of white blood cell degeneration to be evaluated and, when bowel rupture has occurred, mixed bacterial populations and plant material to be assessed.

Examination of the peritoneal fluid, while not a definitive diagnostic test, is a sensitive indicator of bowel injury and provides valuable information regarding the degree of intestinal degeneration. It must be remembered that normal peritoneal fluid may be obtained by abdominocentesis even when an established strangulation obstruction is present due to compartmentalization – for example, in horses with intussusceptions or herniation into the chest, lesser omental bursa or vaginal sac.

Changes in peritoneal fluid associated with peritonitis and non-strangulating infarctions are usually present at the onset of clinical signs. Since these signs are often vague and not very helpful, identification of the abnormal peritoneal fluid avoids delay in instituting the appropriate therapy. Peritoneal fluid from a case of peritonitis is usually milky in appearance due to the high number of white blood cells and few red blood cells. Fluid from cases of non-strangulating infarction varies considerably in its appearance generally appearing opaque due to protein and white blood cells but also, on occasions, red-tinged due to the presence of red blood cells.

Peritoneal fluid samples taken after surgery or caecal decompression have an increase in protein and WBC counts, which persist for a few days.

Complications

Abdominocentesis is, on the whole, a safe technique. Accidental penetration of distended gut with a needle results in no significant contamination of the peritoneal cavity. Evidence of such punctures in the form of a small haemorrhagic spot in the gut wall is seen when the intestine is examined at laparotomy. Of greater worry are partial thickness lacerations due to movement of the needle in an arc across the surface of the distended, fluid-filled small intestine. On very rare occasions, full thickness lacerations may lead to fatal contamination. Therefore, if rectal examination reveals severe small bowel dilatation, paracentesis should be performed with extreme caution, if at all. Similarly, use of a blunt-tipped cannula rather than a needle is recommended in foals to avoid lacerating the thin-walled intestine.

Infection

Temperature

The rectal temperature should be taken routinely during examination of the colic case before rectal examination has been performed. The majority of cases have rectal temperatures within the normal range. Slight elevations may occur due to physical exertion or high environmental temperatures, but significant increases to 38.9°C (102.0°F) or above only occur in response to infections such as Salmonella, anterior enteritis and Ptomac fever. A total and differential WBC count can be useful in these cases.

CBC

The CBC is particularly useful in identifying an acute leucopenia (< 3000 cells/μl), indicating Salmonellosis, Potomac fever or Gram-negative sepsis or endotoxaemia, or a leucocytosis, as might be seen with anterior enteritis or a mesenteric abscess. With the exception of the true monocytosis seen with Potomac fever, a differential WBC count is often not helpful in making a diagnosis.

Summary

The signs of colic are summarized in Table 2.4.

Laboratory examinations

Hydration shock

Packed cell volume (PCV) and total plasma protein are the most commonly used laboratory values in the assessment of hydration, and should always be considered together. PCV is likely to increase in the face of hypovolaemia and dehydration caused by loss of extracellular and intracellular fluid, but *not* blood. Enormous individual variations call for care in interpretation of single samples. Albumin is responsible for about 65 per cent of colloid osmatic pressure. Total protein should increase in

Table 2.4 Physical examination

*Pain	intensity, continuous or intermittent
Bodily condition	signs of trauma, sweating, muscular tremors
*Cardiovascular status	
	heart rate
	pulse quality
	mucus membrane colour
	capillary refill time
	packed cell volume
	total protein
	respiratory rate
	temperature
Abdominal examination	
	?distension, 'guarding'
	inguinal/scrotal region
	auscultation
	*rectal examination
	*nasogastric intubation
	abdominocentesis

*most important criteria

the face of hypovolaemia, but it is important to be aware that hypoproteinaemia can obscure the interpretation of hypovolaemia. A rapid loss of protein is often caused by loss into the peritoneum due to peritonitis or intestinal infarction. Another cause of disparity between the protein and PCV is splenic contraction, which results in an increase in PCV without a concurrent rise in TP. This is often quite dramatic after correction of left dorsal displacement of the large colon.

Fluid electrolyte balance

Electrolyte balance

Electrolyte and acid–base balance are involved with normal intestinal motility, and must be kept in balance during the treatment period. Since there are no clinical parameters that will reliably predict derangements in electrolytes, it is necessary to determine electrolyte values. Sodium, potassium and chloride and calcium may be increased or decreased in response to a variety of disease conditions. Knowledge of electrolyte values is necessary to allow the appropriate fluid to be selected to meet the individual needs of each patient.

Sodium is primarily an extracellular ion, and thereby provides information on relative deficits of water and electrolytes in the extracellular fluid space. To determine the sodium deficit, the following formula is used:

$$\{Na \; normal \; (mEq/l) \times Na \; measure \; (mEq/l)\} \times body \; weight \; (kg) \times 0.3 = Na \; deficit \; (mEq/l)$$

In contrast, potassium is primarily an intracellular ion. Therefore, levels measured in serum or plasma may not be completely representative of the status of intracellular potassium.

Hypokalaemia may occur in horses with colic, from loss of potassium into the lumen of distended bowel. Some horses may have a total body deficit of potassium, but maintain a normal serum K^+, particularly when metabolic acidosis is present or after urine production has ceased. Failure to correlate the serum potassium level with the acid–base status may result in a tremendous underestimation of the total body potassium deficit. Hypokalaemia in the presence of acidosis represents a severe intracellular potassium deficit.

The following formula is used to determine the potassium deficit:

$$\{K^+ \; desired \; (mEq/l) \times K \; measured \; (mEq/l)\} \times bodyweight \; (kg) \times 0.3 = K^+ \; deficit \; (mEq/l)$$

Calcium is often lowered acutely in colic cases, and may be responsible for the lack of intestinal motility. Calcium is useful in maintaining cardiac contractility, and may be necessary as an intravenous drip prior to and during anaesthesia.

Acid–base balance

The metabolic status of horses with colic varies from severe alkalosis to severe acidosis. Since gastrointestinal disease often causes hypovolaemia, reduced tissue perfusion and an increased metabolic rate, derangements in the acid–base status usually result in a metabolic acidosis. The metabolic status cannot be determined by history alone without laboratory tests. For example, a horse with excessive gastric reflux should have a metabolic alkalosis but, if hypovolaemia is severe, the animal may have a normal metabolic status or may have progressed to a metabolic acidosis.

The bicarbonate deficit and replacement requirements are based on the volume of extracellular fluid, body weight and base deficit as determined by venous or arterial blood gas analysis according to the following formula:

Body weight (kg) × base deficit (mEq/l) × 0.3 = bicarbonate deficit (mEq/l)

Ancillary examinations

Radiology

Radiography of the animal with colic has very limited application in the adult horse due to its size and the volume of ingesta in its large intestine. Although penetration may be possible, scattered radiation precludes a clear image and increases the risks to personnel. It is of value in demonstrating the presence of enteroliths and in assessing gastric emptying. However, radiography is of greater value in foals and immature horses, and goes some way to compensating for the clinician's inability to carry out rectal examination in these young animals. Intestinal distension can clearly be seen on standing lateral radiographs, and obstructions due to meconium sand or congenital atresia can often be identified aided by the use of contrast studies.

Ultrasonography

Ultrasonography allows imaging of certain soft tissues associated with the alimentary system, but in many cases excessive gas normally present in the intestine prevents ultrasound penetration. The technique is often limited to evaluating structures within 1–25 cm, and optimally 15 cm, of the abdominal wall. A sector scan head is preferable to a linear scan head. The scan head frequency used depends on the size of the animal and the depths of the structure to be examined. Increasing the scan head frequency improves the resolution, but decreases the depth of penetration. Thus, a frequency of 5.0–7.5 MHz may be sufficient for examination of the foal abdomen, whereas a frequency of 2.0–5.0 MHz is usually required to examine abdominal viscera in adults. It is preferable to clip the site to be examined, but this may not be necessary if the coat is short and the hair is wetted with alcohol.

Several abnormalities may be detected by ultrasonography, including diaphragmatic hernia, dorsal displacement of the colon over the nephrosplenic ligament, peritoneal effusions and abdominal abscesses. In horses with dorsal displacement of the colon into the nephrosplenic space, scanning with a 2.5 MHz sector scanner demonstrates a gas-filled viscus dorsal to the spleen and enveloping its dorsal aspect. A small number of false negative results do occur.

Incarcerated small intestine, with its thickened hypoechoic wall and fluid distension of its lumen, may be identified, for example, in the right dorsal quadrant when herniation has occurred from left to right through the epiploic foramen. The target or bull's eye appearance of small intestinal intussusceptions is characteristic. Two concentric rings can be seen, with a circular inner area or central echogenic core.

Meconium or ascarid impactions may be imaged as intraluminal masses facilitated by fluid distension proximally. Scans *per rectum* can be used to examine the cranial mesenteric artery, mesenteric abscesses and caecal intussusceptions, and to determine the amount of distension and wall thickness of affected small intestine. The keys to an effective use of ultrasonography are a sound knowledge of the anatomy of the abdominal viscera, particularly within 20 cm of the body wall, and frequent use of the diagnostic tool.

Endoscopy

The availability of specialized equipment has expanded the use of this procedure in evaluating the equine alimentary tract. A fibre-optic or video endoscope of 10 mm or less in outer diameter can be passed along the ventral meatus of foals as well as adults. A length of 110 cm is sufficient to reach the stomach of foals, but 200 cm is required to examine the stomachs of yearlings and adults and 275–300 cm to view the duodenum. Food must be withheld for 12 hours prior to gastroscopy for total visualization of the stomach, but even so some ingesta may remain, making evaluation of the glandular stomach and pylorus difficult. Once the stomach is entered, the endoscope usually passes along the greater curvature. The margo plicatis is readily recognized. By bending the tip of the scope 90–180°, the cardia can be examined. Examination of the oesophagus is facilitated by distending it with air, allowing lesions caused by non-steroidal anti-inflammatory drugs or the linear ulcerations associated with grass sickness to be seen.

Faecal examination

Observations of the consistency and colour of the faeces, the presence of foreign material such as sand and the presence of parasites should be included.

Cytological examinations are primarily used to evaluate the parasitic burden of the animal. Ova of small and large strongyles, tapeworms, ascarids and *Strongyloides westeri* are the most common. Coccidia are occasionally observed. Testing for faecal occult blood is often unreliable, particularly if a previous rectal examination has caused some bleeding. Although it can be useful in cases of gastric ulceration or ulceration due to non-steroidal anti-inflammatory drugs, most gastric ulcers do not bleed; a negative occult blood does not therefore rule out this problem. Faecal culture is used primarily to detect Salmonella spp. Samples are plated directly onto an appropriate agar–brilliant green or DCA, and as a subculture after placement in selenite broth, which is the most widely used enrichment medium for Salmonella. The increasing incidence of colic in which *Clostridium perfringens* appears to be implicated merits the use of culture techniques aimed at isolating this organism in some horses. Samples are immediately transferred to meat broth and incubated overnight at 37°. Cultures are then plated onto sheep blood agar and incubated in an anaerobic atmosphere. Once a pure culture has been obtained, it is subjected to a series of biochemical tests for final identification of the organism.

Laparoscopy

Laparoscopy may be performed in the standing, sedated animal, but requires feed being withheld for at least 12 and preferably 36 hours, to reduce the size of the caecum and large colon. The laparoscopic sleeve is carefully inserted through a small 2 cm incision in the right or left paralumbar fossa. Allowing air to enter the peritoneal cavity is usually adequate for a routine examination using a 30° angled scope. In a 'normal' horse, identifiable structures that can be seen via a left flank approach include the liver, stomach, spleen, nephrosplenic ligament, inguinal ring, ovary, uterus, rectum, pelvic flexure and small intestine. From the right flank, the duodenum, base of caecum, inguinal ring, ovary, uterus and rectum can be examined. Intestinal distension is a serious limitation, and is a major problem in horses with colic due to the risk of puncture and the masking of lesions. Negative findings are common if one is merely exploring the abdomen for some suspected abnormality. Laparoscopy should always be preceded by a careful physical examination and abdominal palpation *per rectum*. A primary indication for laparoscopy is a palpable abdominal mass that requires further characterization.

Summary of possible causes of colic

Table 2.5 gives a brief summary of the signs and possible diagnoses for horses suffering from colic.

The decision for surgery

Recognition of the case requiring surgery

Making the decision to operate on a horse exhibiting signs of abdominal pain should, theoretically, be straightforward. Either the patient has a life-threatening intestinal obstruction or it does not. Theoretically, the animal requiring surgery is in pain, has distended intestine palpable on rectal examination, has abnormal characteristics to its peritoneal fluid, few or no intestinal sounds on auscultation and, in the case of obstruction of the small intestine, significant volumes of fluid should be retrievable by nasogastric intubation. Unfortunately, the theoretical and real worlds do not always coincide. Such is often the case with equine colic, where the type of obstruction, its location and severity and the interval that has

Table 2.5 Signs and possible diagnoses for horses suffering from colic

Pain	None		Mild	Severe
	Enteritis		Ileus	Strangulation
	Ileus		Obstruction	Obstruction
			Peritonitis	Enteritis
Temperature	Normal		Fever	
	Ileus		Enteritis	
	Obstruction		Peritonitis	
	Strangulation			
Heart rate	Normal		Increased	
	Ileus		Obstruction	
	Peritonitis		Strangulation	
			Peritonitis	
			Enteritis	
Gastric reflus	None		Present	
	Large colon obstruction		Gastric dilation	
	Small colon obstruction		SI obstruction	
	Colitis		Strangulation	
	Peritonitis		SI enteritis	
			Grass sickness	
Rectal examination	Normal		Abnormal	
	Peritonitis		Obstruction	
	Large colon enteritis		Strangulation	
			SI enteritis	
			Gastrointestinal rupture	
White blood cell count	Normal		Increased/decreased	
	Ileus		Peritonitis	
	Obstruction		Enteritis	
	Strangulation		Abscess	
Peritoneal fluid	Normal		Increased	
	Ileus		Obstruction	
	Large colon enteritis		Strangulation	
			Peritonitis	
			SI enteritis	

elapsed since it occurred make for tremendous variation in the clinical signs at presentation.

Although at many referral centres the facilities are available for a battery of laboratory tests, which allow accurate assessment of the animals' haematologic and metabolic status, on the whole these are of assistance in evaluating pre-operative preparation and prognosis. They very seldom help the surgeon decide which horse needs surgical intervention. Consequently, at such institutions (as in the field) the decision is predominantly based on the result of the physical examination.

Surgical intervention is indicated under the following circumstances:

1. When the exact cause of the colic can be diagnosed and the obstructing lesion requires surgery for its correction.

2. When there is no exact diagnosis, but there is sufficient evidence to indicate that surgery is the only means of saving the animal's life.
3. When animals with recurrent colic over a period of days or weeks are suspected of having partial obstruction due to intussusception, neoplasia, adhesions etc.

History and signalment   Several components of the history and signalment may help the surgeon to decide whether or not surgery is indicated. For instance, age- and sex-related conditions must be borne in mind. Obstructive conditions involving the distal colon or rectum and defects in the urinary tract occur commonly in neonatal foals. Ileal or ileocaecal intussusceptions tend to occur in horses younger than 18 months of age and, to emphasize the point further, epiploic foramen entrapments generally occur in horses older than 8 years and pedunculated lipomas cause problems in horses over 12 years of age.

Colonic torsions are most common in mares which have foaled within the previous 60 days, while inguinal hernias in stallions are frequently associated with a history of recently covering a mare or exercise.

Pain   Pain is an important determinant for surgery, and should always be considered. In many clinical situations, surgical exploration of the abdominal cavity is undertaken for no other reason than the presence of severe unrelenting pain. In most of these cases, something of surgical importance is found in the abdomen and the patient benefits from the early intervention.

Shock   Progressive cardiovascular deterioration is another important determinant for surgery. A progressively increasing heart rate, weakening pulse, congestion of mucus membranes, increased PCV and extended LRT are evidence of impending circulatory collapse. These changes are most rapid and severe in horses with ischaemic gut, particularly those with 360° large colon torsion and strangulation obstruction of considerable lengths of small intestine. They occur more slowly in horses with complete non-strangulating obstruction of the small intestine, such as ileal impaction, while conditions such as caeco-caecal intussusception may result in very little alteration in cardiovascular parameters even when they have been in existence for several days. Cases of enteritis that do not require surgery can also show signs of severe shock. In these cases, signs of shock must be carefully evaluated in lieu of other physical findings when considering the need for surgery.

Physical examination features

Rectal examination
As indicated previously, rectal examination is the single most important part of the clinical work-up of the horse with abdominal disease. The decision for surgery is usually based on the findings at rectal examination

carried out after reviewing the pertinent aspects of the history, particularly the duration of colic, and the rest of the physical examination. In this way, an attempt can be made to predict what should be felt and to compare the findings with these preconceived ideas. For example, a relatively short history of severe abdominal pain in an 18-year-old pony, reflux on passage of a nasogastric tube and minimal abdominal distension should suggest a small intestinal obstruction, probably by a lipoma. Rectal examination should be approached in the expectation of finding gas/fluid-distended loops of small intestine. It must be emphasized that certain conditions may be diagnosed by rectal palpation before the animal becomes severely ill or changes in peritoneal fluid become evident. Consequently, the rectal examination is of paramount importance in identifying such conditions as large colon torsion, colonic displacements, ileocaecal intussusception, ileal impaction and inguinal hernia.

Nasogastric intubation

The presence of volumes of gastric reflux in excess of 3 l is another finding that warrants concern and, in most cases, indicates a surgical problem. However, large volumes of reflux are a feature of proximal enteritis and acute grass sickness, conditions that simulate simple or strangulating obstructions of small intestine with regard to other clinical findings. Whether or not these horses undergo exploratory surgery for confirmation of the diagnosis is based on the surgeon's conclusion about the significance of each sign in consideration of all the others.

Peritoneal fluid sample

While most horses with colic admitted to referral centres have a peritoneal fluid sample taken and analysed, the result is of secondary importance to the rectal findings and the degree of pain in identifying the need for surgery in the majority of cases. However, the results of these analyses often help to identify the horse with gastrointestinal rupture, primary peritonitis and non-strangulating infarction. Whenever possible, horses should be referred for surgery before marked changes in peritoneal fluid have taken place.

Response to treatment   Failure of colic cases to respond to medical therapy, particularly the persistence of severe pain despite analgesic therapy, is a significant indication of the need for surgery. However, the emergence of new potent prostaglandin synthetase inhibitors such as flunixin has complicated the issue. Now, horses having intestinal ischaemia requiring surgical intervention may appear to respond to treatment with such compounds for several hours. For this reason, horses with colic that are given non-steroidal anti-inflammatory drugs should be monitored very closely, and repeated use of these drugs should be avoided. Frequently, signs of colic recur in horses with a serious lesion within 1–2 hours of administration of flunixin, but these signs will be markedly decreased. Therefore, if any sign of discomfort is observed after treatment with a potent analgesic, it is highly probable that the horse has a surgical condition.

Table 2.6 summarizes the criteria for surgical intervention. However, these are only guidelines. Because of the great variation in the type of obstruction, the segment and length of gut involved and the degree of occlusion, some cases will inevitably cause problems in diagnosis. When evidence for and against surgery is evenly balanced, intuition based on clinical experience is often the deciding factor. Veterinarians are encouraged to refer cases for further examination and, if necessary, surgery, rather than wait until they are certain of their diagnosis. This inevitably results in some horses and owners making what might be considered to be unnecessary journeys if further evaluation at the referral centre shows that surgery is unnecessary but, more importantly, it reduces the number of horses which do not survive to make the return journey.

The key to success in colic surgery is being able to make the decision to perform surgery as early as possible. If this can be done, all parties – including the owner of the horse, the referring veterinarian and the surgeon – will be pleased with the outcome.

Preparation of a horse for transport to a surgical facility

The following measures should be taken in preparation for transport of the horse:

1. Decompress the horse's stomach and, if the length of journey merits it, leave the nastogastric tube in place and tape it to the head collar.
2. Administer an analgesic. If it is clear that surgery is necessary and a strangulation obstruction is suspected, flunixin is the drug of choice because, in addition to relieving pain, it will counter the effects of endotoxaemia. Detomidine is a satisfactory alternative, providing sedation and analgesia.

Table 2.6 Summary of criteria for surgical intervention

Positive rectal findings identifying a specific surgical problem or indicating acute abdominal disease

Severe unrelenting pain with no, or only a short-term, response to analgesics

Progressive cardiovascular deterioration – pulse rate increasing progressively and weakening: PCV. 50, injected mucus membranes and increased capillary refill time

Positive paracentesis findings – increased protein, red blood cells and white blood cells

Progressive reduction in intestinal motility – gastric reflux of alkaline bile-stained fluid

Increasing, life-threatening distension

---

3. If the horse is in shock, electrolytes may be given to improve circulating blood volume while awaiting arrival of transport, but departure to the surgical centre should not be delayed for the purpose of administering the large volumes necessary to make any significant impression on the packed cell volume. On arrival at the centre, a rapid improvement in the cardiovascular status of severely shocked horses can be achieved by administration of 2.5 l of hypertonic saline. This is not an option prior to referral, because a large volume of isotonic fluid must be administered within 2 hours of the hypertonic solution.
4. Administer a broad-spectrum antibiotic.
5. Rug the horse up and bandage its limbs.
6. Provide a detailed report of the treatment administered prior to referral.
7. Provide the owner with accurate directions how to get to the hospital.

The possibility of gastric rupture having occurred in any horses suspected of having gastric dilation should always be borne in mind, particularly if there is sudden cessation of overt pain followed by rapid progressive cardiovascular deterioration. Retrieval of gas and no fluid or only a small volume of fluid on passing a nasogastric tube in a horse which has numerous loops of distended small intestinal palpable on rectal examination should cause suspicion of gastric rupture. A peritoneal tap will reveal dark brown fluid in which particles of food may be identified. Further evidence of abdominal catastrophe is obtained where, on rectal examination, the serosal surfaces of the intestine are felt to be rough due to adherent particles of digesta, and free gas in the abdominal cavity makes it surprisingly easy to pass a hand between loops of distended small intestine.

A significant number of horses sent to referral centres are found on arrival to have gastric rupture. While in some cases this may have happened in transit, in others it will have occurred before the horse was loaded. It is imperative that gastric rupture is diagnosed promptly and that the horse is euthanased immediately to avoid the unnecessary suffering which a pointless journey would entail.

3

Medical treatments

Analgesia

The main aims in treating the patient with colic are to relieve pain, treat dehydration and shock, and restore normal transit of ingesta. The primary treatments to relieve pain are decompression of the stomach and intestines, and administration of analgesics. Treating dehydration and shock, which can accompany all but the mildest cases of colic, requires administration of intravenous fluids and, in some cases, agents that combat endotoxaemia. Restoring intestinal transit can be challenging and, in some cases, can be aided by pharmacologic treatments.

Decompression

A primary method of relieving pain is by decompression of the distended stomach or intestine. Nasogastric intubation can help relieve gastric tympany or remove gastrointestinal reflux due to a small intestinal obstruction or ileus. The tube can be left in place for chronic decompression after surgery or for cases of proximal enteritis, but should be checked routinely as stomach pressure may not force the fluid through the tube, even with massive distension. Horses with gastric dilatation have suffered stomach rupture, even after the recent passage of a stomach tube or with a stomach tube left in place for passive decompression. In all cases, an attempt to start a siphon should be made by filling the tube with water and then lowering the end of the tube below the level of the stomach (see Chapter 2). In those cases suspected of having chronic fluid accumulation, monitoring stomach distension every 3 hours is recommended.

The other site at which gaseous pressure can be relieved by decompression is the caecum. This can resolve a primary caecal tympany or help relieve gas build-up from a large colon or small colon obstruction. Decompression of large colon distension is more difficult, and is seldom recommended unless the manoeuvre can be guided *per rectum*. It is rare that decompression is helpful in relieving colon tympany and frequently, when the colon is distended enough to require decompression, a surgical lesion is present. Decompression of the caecum is done in the right paralumbar fossa midway between the last rib and the ventral prominence of the tuber coxae. A 12.5–15 cm (5–6 in) 14–16 gauge needle or catheter over a needle is used. The caecal trochar (which is 10–12 gauge) should not be used as it can result in a tear in the caecum, which can later leak ingesta into the peritoneal cavity. The skin should be surgically prepared, and aseptic technique used to place the needle. The needle is pushed through the flank into the caecum by keeping the needle perpendicular to the skin. The landmarks should be used carefully so as to avoid placing the needle too high in the caecum. Suction is helpful for rapid reduction of caecal tympany. A concurrent rectal examination can help push gas into the caecal base, and facilitate removing as much as possible. Once the gas is removed, saline should be infused through the needle as it is pulled out of the caecum and through the body wall to avoid leaving a tract of contaminated material. Once the caecum is empty, a thorough rectal examination is repeated to determine if the tympany is primary or secondary to another condition.

Systemic analgesics

Systemic analgesics are the most common way to control colic. Although there is anecdotal information and have been clinical trials reporting evidence of efficacy of these compounds, the experimental studies that have been done in horses to provide information about the usefulness of drugs for specific types of pain have predominately used a distension model to emulate visceral pain. When tested, flunixin meglumine (flunixin), xylazine, detomidine and butorphanol were the only drugs which gave long-term and dependable results in controlling severe pain from caecal distension (Kalpravidh, 1984; Lowe, 1978; Lowe and Hilfiger, 1984, 1986a, 1986b; Muir and Robertson, 1985; Muir *et al.*, 1982).

NSAIDs

One of the most useful groups of analgesics for both surgical and non-surgical disease is the non-steroidal anti-inflammatory drugs (NSAIDs). These drugs block the enzyme cyclo-oxygenase, thereby decreasing the production of prostaglandins by blocking cyclo-oxygenase in the arachidonic acid cascade. Prostaglandin E_2 and I_2 are known to sensitize nerve endings to pain, and are possibly responsible for amplification of pain during bowel distension, ischaemia and inflammation. Prostaglandin F_{2a} will induce smooth muscular contraction and can cause vasoconstriction (Masri *et al.*, 1985). Both PGE_2 and PGF_{2a} cause longitudinal muscle contraction, whereas circular muscle contracts in response to PGF_{2a}. PGE_2 increases caused by endotoxaemia are associated with intestinal ileus. Thromboxane, another product of the arachidonic cascade, can cause marked vasoconstriction with subsequent ischaemia, resulting in pain. The effect of prostaglandins during equine intestinal disease is not fully understood. However, there is a favourable response during colic after administration of drugs that inhibit their formation (Moore *et al.*, 1981).

Flunixin is the most effective of the NSAIDs used to treat acute abdominal disease in the horse, and has been shown to block the production of the prostaglandins, specifically thromboxane and prostacyclin, for 8–12 hours after a single dose. Advantages of this therapy are the maintenance of normal blood flow to the bowel during obstruction (Lowe *et al.*, 1980) and a return of intestinal motility. In cases where a strangulated segment of intestine is suspected, the use of flunixin pre-operatively can be helpful in diminishing the detrimental response due to the endotoxin release (Moore, 1985). After treatment, horses with impactions or peritonitis will have increased comfort (6–8 hours) and a return of borborygmi. Flunixin can obscure the signs of endotoxaemia and distension or strangulation to some degree. The inability to eliminate pain with flunixin suggests a disease exists that requires more than simple medical treatment. For this reason, horses given flunixin should be observed carefully after its administration. If signs of colic return, particularly after a short period, the horse should immediately be suspected of having more than a simple medical colic. The dose of flunixin can sometimes be reduced to a quarter or half of the manufacturer's dose (1.1 mg/kg) in some cases of impaction and enteritis, and post-operatively for suppression of the signs from endotoxaemia (Semrad *et al.*, 1985).

Phenylbutazone is not as good an analgesic for colic as flunixin, and does not inhibit prostaglandin formation as well as or for as long as flunixin (Moore *et al.*, 1986). Its use appears to be more helpful for musculoskeletal problems than for visceral pain, though the reason for this difference is not known. Recent evidence indicates that phenylbutazone is more effective in reducing PGE_2, thereby reversing ileus during endotoxaemia. The dosage response for this is not known, but 1–2 mg/kg has been used.

Dipyrone is another NSAID and is reported to have an antispasmodic effect on bowel because of its inhibition in response to bradykinin. Dipyrone's effectiveness as a true spasmolytic in horses with colic is not confirmed, but there appears to be some inhibition of prostaglandin formation, which can explain its analgesic and spasmolytic effect. It is successfully used for mild colic, but its effect is short-lived (Lowe, 1978) and it is ineffective in treating colic from severe obstruction or strangulation.

Ketoprofen (an analogue of ibuprofen) has been used clinically for treatment of colic. It has been shown to be effective against subclinical endotoxaemia, similar to flunixin, though it is claimed to block lipoxygenase, which reduces the formation of leukotrienes. Gastric ulceration is also said to be less of a risk with this drug, though at low doses this is not considered to be a problem with flunixin. Ketoprofen is reported anecdotally to be less effective as an analgesic than flunixin meglumine. Ketoprofen is able to block leukotriene production, but there is little evidence of clinical benefit to date.

Aspirin can only be administered orally, and has such a short half-life in the horse that it has little efficacy in treating acute abdominal pain. It may be useful in non-strangulating disease by reducing platelet production of thromboxane, thereby reducing platelet aggregation and vasoconstriction. Drugs such as meclofenamic acid and naproxin are also ineffective in treating colic.

Disadvantages of the NSAIDs (particularly phenylbutazone) include the potential for toxicity, causing mucosal ulceration of the gastro-intestinal tract or renal damage (White, 1990a). This is particularly true if they are used orally, for long periods, during periods of dehydration and/or in combination with aminoglycoside antibiotics (Adams and McClure, 1985). Toxicity may be avoided in many cases by reducing the dosage.

Alpha-2 agonists

Several alpha-2 agonists are potent analgesics, and cause muscle relaxation and sedation. This drug group includes xylazine and detomidine, both of which have been used for control of pain in the acute abdomen. The actions appear to be central $alpha_2$ adrenoreceptor stimulation, which modulates the release of norepinephrine and directly inhibits neuronal firing (Virtanen, 1986). This causes sedation, analgesia, bradycardia and, in the horse with colic, relief of pain. Other responses to these drugs are important, as they can affect their use in horses with shock. The heart rate can be markedly reduced by second degree heart block, with heart rates of less than 20 per minute being recorded. This causes a significant reduction in the cardiac output for a short period of time, and may thereby have a detrimental effect on the horse that already has a critical reduction in circulating blood volume. There is also a brief period of vasoconstriction which, in the normal horse, is of minimal concern, but may cause complications in horses where poor tissue perfusion is already occurring due to shock. Alpha-2 agonists reduce the blood flow of an obstructed large intestine and decrease intraluminal pressure (MacKay, 1992). Similarly, in experimental small intestinal ischaemia, xylazine reduced blood flow and increased oxygen utilization. There is a transient increase in urine production, which may complicate dehydration and circulatory shock (Virtanen, 1986).

Xylazine also has potent effects on intestinal motility, and the jejunum and large intestine have less activity for up to 2 hours following a 1.1 mg/kg dose (Adams, 1988). This is a profound effect, giving relief from both somatic and visceral pain caused by distension or strangulation. Xylazine may be indicated to help relax contracting intestine or to help restrain a horse in order to prepare for surgery. Analgesia may only last for 10–30 minutes, or may have minimal effect in cases of severe strangulation such as large colon torsion. In cases of large or small colon impactions it appears beneficial in relieving the spasm of the intestine around the obstructing mass, thereby allowing passage of gas and rehydration of ingesta. This can often be accomplished with doses of 0.1–0.3 mg/kg intravenously. If a prolonged effect is desired, xylazine can be administered intramuscularly at doses of 0.4–2 mg/kg. The lower the dose, the less the risk of untoward reactions. Because of the possible complicating effects of lowered blood flow to the intestine, xylazine should be used only when necessary. Xylazine has been used successfully in horses with various types of intestinal disease, and repeatedly on difficult cases with satisfactory results. In cases of large colon distension or impaction, its use in low doses is helpful in relieving spasm and allowing gas to pass by the obstruction. The short period of ileus is not detrimental, and is often followed by resumption of intestinal transit.

Detomidine is an alpha-2 agonist like xylazine, and is a potent sedative (Lowe and Hilfiger, 1984). It can produce complete cessation of colic for up to 3 hours and, during experimental caecal distension, provided mean analgesia of 45 and 105 minutes at 20 µg/kg and 40 µg/kg respectively. Horses stand with their heads lowered and are reluctant to move. Its action is centrally mediated, similar to that of xylazine but with a much longer duration (Lowe and Hilfiger, 1986). Second degree heart blocks are common, it will reduce intestinal motility as with xylazine, and it can obscure signs of pain that might help the clinician diagnose the cause of the colic. Since this is such a potent drug, any signs of colic observed within an hour of administration are an indication that severe disease is present and the horse may require surgery. When used, cases should be monitored appropriately.

Both xylazine and detomidine are potent sedatives. Their use facilitates rectal examination by providing restraint and some relaxation of the rectum and abdominal cavity. Care should be taken when initiating the rectal examination, as horses can suddenly kick when first touched. Both drugs have been used as pre-anaesthetics in critical cases without compromising the patient during general anaesthesia.

Opioids

The pure opioid agonists such as morphine and oxymorphone are potent analgesics, but they can cause excitation in the horse unless used in combination with drugs such as xylazine. Morphine is known to reduce progressive motility of the small intestine and colon, while potentially increasing mixing movements and increasing sphincter tone (Adams *et al.*, 1984; Kalpravidh, 1984). This can increase transit time. The disadvantages of morphine and oxymorphone in the horse with abdominal disease are sufficient to discourage their use (Pippi and Lumb, 1979).

Meperidine is an opioid agonist with few side effects in the horse (Lowe, 1978). Analgesia is slight and variable, depending on the source of pain. It does not provide long-term analgesia. Used repeatedly, it can potentiate obstruction due to impaction by reducing progressive motility in the colons (Adams *et al.*, 1984). Compared with the other opiate agonists, when used for visceral pain, it was similar to oxymorphone and pentazocine in effect over time (Pippi and Lumb, 1979).

Butorphanol is a partial agonist and antagonist that gives the best pain relief with the least side effects seen with opioids (Muir *et al.*, 1982). It can also be used in combination with xylazine. The dosage can vary from 0.05–0.1 mg/kg, the higher dosage being necessary for the most severe colic. Exceeding 0.2 mg/kg may cause an increase in heart rate, systolic blood pressure and excitation in horses (Robertson *et al.*, 1981). Butorphanol reduces small intestinal motility, yet has minimal effect on pelvic flexure activity (Sojka *et al.*, 1988). The drug is potent enough to stop colic due to severe intestinal disease for short periods of time, though the pain from large colon torsion and small intestinal volvulus may not be altered. Butorphanol does not affect the cardiovascular system except at higher doses, and can therefore be administered to the horse suffering from circulatory shock and as part of a pre-anaesthetic protocol. Repeated use has the risk of increasing transit time and causing impaction formation, as seen with other opiate-like drugs. Overdosage can be partially reversed with equal doses of naloxone.

Pentazocine is a partial agonist that has some analgesic effect in horses with colic. Similarly to other opioids, it appears to work centrally. It provides relatively weak analgesia for colic, providing relief for only minutes during severe episodes of pain (Lowe, 1978; Sojka *et al.*, 1988). It may have some beneficial effect when combined with xylazine. Its side effects at the doses recommended by the manufacturer are minimal. When the dosage is increased, central excitatory effects are possible.

Spasmolytics

Spasmolytic drugs can indirectly provide analgesia by reducing spasms of the intestine (Adams *et al.*, 1984). Increased frequency of intestinal contractions or spasms occurs oral to an intraluminal obstruction such as an impaction. Spasmolytic drugs include cholinergic blockers such as atropine, which can cause colic when administered to the normal horse by causing ileus and secondary tympany (Ducharme and Fubini, 1983). Though not recommended, atropine has been used to treat colic and is effective by relaxing the intestinal wall and preventing intestinal contractions. The effect can unfortunately extend from several hours to several days, allowing tympany and complicating the initial problem with ileus (Ducharme and Fubini, 1983). The administration of this treatment was once a common practice in horse owners, who gave Bell's solution, an oral tonic containing belladonna. Its use for the equine acute abdomen is contraindicated.

The combination of scopolamine and para-aminophenol derivative (dipyrone) known as Buscopan® is popular in Europe for treatment of colic, specifically for colic due to impactions (Davies and Gerring, 1983). Scopolamine has shorter-acting muscarinic cholinergic blocking effects compared to atropine, and is effective in relaxing the bowel wall to prevent contraction. The drug can be detrimental in horses with ileus, where inhibition of motility causes tympany and complicates the abdominal stasis already present. This drug is useful for most mild colic and impactions. Similarly to xylazine detomidine, the relaxation afforded to the intestine appears beneficial in relieving pain and eventually restoring normal motility.

Miscellaneous sedatives

Diazepam is a sedative which, though not classified as an analgesic, can be used to help control pain from gastric ulceration in the foal. Used at a dosage of 0.05–0.1 mg/kg, diazepam stops the outward appearance of pain. Foals will stop grinding their teeth and colic will cease. The mechanism for the pain relief is not known.

Chloral hydrate, another sedative, works centrally and has minimal effects on the cardiac output or intestinal motility at the lower doses (40–60 mg/kg) used for sedation and relief of pain. It is most effective for treatment of intestinal impactions, and acts by reducing the horses activity and hence propensity to injure itself. Though there seem to be few adverse effects, it has not been shown to have the same relaxing effect on the bowel and there appears to be no reduction in the mediators of pain as seen with the NSAIDs. Chloral hydrate, therefore, is no longer recommended for common colic problems. If used, it is given intravenously and is titrated to effect after the initial dose. It should be given by catheter since it is extremely irritating and can cause severe phlebitis or perivascular necrosis if not administered properly. Chloral hydrate is an anaesthetic and, if overdosed, can produce weakness, recumbency and eventually reduced cardiac output. Its use should be restricted to reduction of pain from a known problem such as an impaction, where the object is to reduce physical activity and anxiety. The drug should not be used without a diagnosis, but rather as an adjunct to other treatments. Alternative drugs are superior in reducing pain in most horses.

Hydration

Hydration of the acute abdominal patient can be the most important treatment, and often determines success or failure in horses with shock. Hydration is usually accomplished with balanced electrolyte solutions such as Ringer's, lactated Ringer's or acetated Ringer's solutions. The greatest need is to replace water. Therefore, sodium replacement with the appropriate solution is needed to maintain the water in the extracellular fluid (ECF) space without sacrificing potassium levels during long-term fluid administration. The level of dehydration is determined by clinical signs of capillary refill, skin turgor, the packed cell volume (PCV) and total protein (TP). This is done by estimating the water loss as a percentage of the body weight or the percentage of the blood or ECF change. An estimate can be calculated from the PCV and TP as follows:

$$\frac{(\text{measured PCV or TP}) - (\text{normal PCV or TP}) \times 100}{(\text{normal PCV or TP})}$$

$$= \text{percentage change in PCV or TP}$$

This percentage change represents the change in the blood or the ECF volume from normal. The calculated percentage multiplied by the blood volume (7 per cent of the body weight in kg = litres of blood) is the estimated amount of fluid that needs to be replaced immediately to provide an adequate circulatory volume; an estimate which is critical for the horse requiring surgery. The same estimate using the ECF volume (30 per cent of the body weight in kg = litres of ECF) calculates the total replacement required for rehydration of the ECF space (White, 1990b).

The effects of dehydration should not be underestimated as a cause or sequela of colic. Horses with slight intestinal distension and ileus with accompanying pain often respond immediately after simple fluid replacement. Intravenous fluid administration has also been helpful in increasing the available fluid for intestinal secretion. The constant secretion of the intestinal tract provides the needed water to soften an impacted food mass. This 'over-hydration' technique can be used as a primary treatment for pelvic flexure and caecal impactions. It should be used rather than repeated administration of oral cathartics in refractory cases.

The goal of over-hydration is to maintain a slightly increased circulating water volume, which will equilibrate with the extracellular space. This equilibration causes secretion into the bowel, particularly at sites of intestinal distension where secretion is initiated by the increase in the capillary filtration. The fluid can be administered intravenously over a 24-hour period, or as a bolus. Use of boluses of fluid should be avoided in horses in shock.

The replacement fluid needs to be balanced, supplying sodium and chloride with adequate potassium replacement. The over-hydration effect is monitored by repeated measurement of the PCV and plasma protein values (every 6 hours). By regulating the chronic intravenous fluid administration to keep the plasma protein at 5.0–5.5 g/dl (normal 6.5 g/dl), a state of over-hydration will be maintained with adequate fluid available to help intestinal secretion. This normally requires a fluid administration rate of 2–4 l per hour, double or triple maintenance requirements. When a bolus of fluids is used, 20 l in 1–2 hours is usually sufficient to lower the plasma protein concentration.

This technique has been successful in softening and resolving caecal and large colon impactions already 5–7 days old and resistant to therapy (Dabareiner and White, 1995). In all cases, the peritoneal fluid should be monitored for evidence of bowel degeneration. Normally, analgesia will not be required during the majority of this therapy. Flunixin meglumine is used at a quarter to half the recommended dose, and xylazine (0.2–0.4 mg/kg) is used when required for periods of pain. If pain can not be controlled, a massive impaction or another lesion is usually present and exploratory surgery is indicated.

Massive fluid administration may be required for enteritis causing secretory diarrhoea and shock. The intensive care and monitoring required for this treatment is not discussed here. If protein is being lost by the intestine or the kidney or into the peritoneal cavity, the protein level will decrease in the face of dehydration. Once this protein level reaches 4.0 g/dl, plasma administration is helpful in maintaining normal vascular osmotic pressure and the vascular volume. Normally, a minimum of 10 l of plasma is required to increase plasma protein levels.

In cases of severe dehydration, including those of endotoxic shock, horses can be treated with hypertonic saline as an emergency measure to restore circulating volume. A 7.5 per cent saline solution is administered at 4–5 ml/kg as rapidly as possible. This quickly draws water from the extracellular and intracellular spaces into the vascular space. This will improve perfusion and lower the heart rate, but it must be followed with adequate replacement fluids to help restore hydration. Hypertonic saline is very useful in resuscitating horses in severe shock, and its use should be reserved for such cases.

Endotoxic shock

The horse with a compromised intestine is at risk of absorbing endotoxin into the blood stream. Experimental endotoxaemia from 0.001 to 0.01

μg/kg causes colic, diarrhoea, poor peripheral perfusion, lactic acidosis, leucopenia and venous pooling (Clark and Moore, 1989; Moore, 1990). Higher doses cause death as a result of circulatory shock. Research has provided some interesting insight into how endotoxin causes shock in both laboratory animals and the horse.

Pathogenesis

Endotoxin, a lipopolysaccharide, is a toxin that must interact with the immune system to cause shock. Key to endotoxin activity is the macrophage. Macrophages, which have endotoxin receptors, produce numerous cytokines (tumour necrosis factor, and interleukins) in response to endotoxin (Moore, 1990). The cytokines in turn cause other cells to release mediators, including prostacyclin, thromboxane, platelet activating factor, reactive oxygen species, proteases, histamine serotonin and leukotrienes (see Fig. 3.1).

A direct action of endotoxin is its interaction with complement, causing activation of complement and production of bradykinin. Tumour necrosis factor initiates much of the damage to cell membranes; specifically, endothelial cells cause a cascade of events, including vascular and haemostatic effects. Cell membrane disruption causes breakdown of arachidonic acid, initiating the prostaglandin cascade and causing even

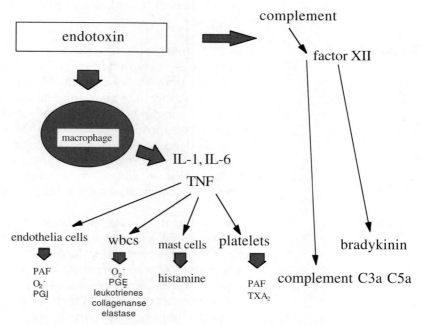

Figure 3.1 Endotoxin attaches to receptors on the macrophage, stimulating cytokine secretion. Interleukin 1, 6 and tumour necrosis factor modulate the response of other cells to produce platelet-activating factor, prostaglandins, superoxide radicals, histamine and proteases. Endotoxin directly stimulates complement to produce C3a and C5a, and activation of Factor XII causes bradykinin production (MacKay, 1992).

further signs of shock, including vasoconstriction of the pulmonary vasculature, vasodilatation of the intestinal vasculature, depression of cardiac output, coagulopathy and, eventually, organ failure (MacKay, 1992).

Endotoxin causes fever by stimulation of TNF and IL-1, which act on the central nervous system. Neutropenia is caused by activation of neutrophils by TNF and leukotriene B4 initiating the adhesion of neutrophils to endothelial cells. Damaged endothelial cells allow migration of neutrophils through the vasculature. Pulmonary hypertension is one of the hallmarks of acute endotoxaemia and is the result of damage to the pulmonary endothelial cells, which causes a 'shock lung' (Moore *et al.*, 1981). The response is increased respiratory rate and poor oxygenation of blood passing through the lung. Systemic blood pressure initially increases in response to vasoconstriction, but soon hypotension is observed as vascular resistance, myocardial depression and reduced plasma volume occur. Coagulability increases by activation of the intrinsic pathway. There is also increased procoagulant activity by endothelial cells and macrophages. Thrombomodulin is reduced by the effect of TNF on the endothelial cells, allowing local coagulopathy. Consumptive coagulopathy leads to diffuse intravascular coagulation (DIC), but this is normally at an irreversible stage of shock. The chief effect of endotoxaemia is a reduction of peripheral perfusion. Hypoxaemia is profound, due to poor oxygen extraction and utilization in the tissues.

Clinical signs

Signs of endotoxaemia include depression, colic, initial periods of loose stool, cyanosis, increased heart and respiratory rates, and fever (Clarke and Moore, 1989; Moore *et al.*, 1981). As shock progresses, hypotension becomes evident by the poor pulse quality, cyanosis (with a cyanotic line around the gingiva), sweating, and cold extremities. Intestinal borborygmi cease during endotoxaemia (Moore, 1990). Laboratory values that help identify shock – and specifically endotoxic shock – include increased PCV, neutropenia in the first 3–4 hours followed by a toxic left shift, lactic acidosis and reduced platelet numbers, and prolongation of prothrombin or activated partial thromboplastin times.

Treatment

The basis of treating endotoxic shock is restoration of circulatory volume. Normally, rapid infusion of a balanced electrolyte solution, such as lactated Ringer's or acetated Ringer's, will improve perfusion. In cases where perfusion is so poor that normal solutions may take too long to provide adequate perfusion, use of hypertonic saline solution may help in immediate resuscitation. When 7 or 8 per cent saline solutions (1–3 l) are rapidly infused, water drawn into the circulation increases blood pressure and cardiac output, helping to sustain the animal until adequate balanced electrolyte solutions can be administered.

Anti-endotoxin antiserum has recently been advocated as a therapy for endotoxaemia. However, there are still mixed reports about the success of antiserum or endotoxin vaccine in protecting against endotoxaemia.

Horses vaccinated with an antigen from the core portion of the lipopolysaccharide of the J-5 mutant *E. coli* were not protected against sublethal endotoxaemia in one study, but clinical reports indicate some benefit (Spier *et al.*, 1989). The use of a methylated Salmonella endotoxin with adjuvant has been found to be valuable when used as a vaccine. The hyperimmune serum from horses vaccinated with this salmonella endotoxin has also been shown to prevent the development of laminitis after experimental carbohydrate overload, and protect against a sublethal intravenous endotoxin challenge. This therapy has also been tested in horses with colic and suspected endotoxaemia. The antiserum appeared to improve the survival rate in these horses (Garner *et al.*, 1985). In clinical cases, the antiserum produced from horses vaccinated with the J-5 *E. coli* or methylated salmonella may be helpful in preventing the ongoing effects of endotoxaemia which occur from continued bowel injury. Horses having endotoxic reactions, with cyanotic mucous membranes, dehydration, increased heart rates and ileus, will often respond rapidly after antiserum administration. Horses have occasionally had physical reactions to rapid administration of the methylated salmonella antiserum. This problem may be avoided by reducing the administration rate, diluting the antiserum or heating the antiserum to at least room temperature prior to administration. Administration of antiserum is recommended in any horse where damaged intestine could produce endotoxaemia. The earlier treatment is started, the better the chance of reducing the effects of endotoxin.

Plasma without antibodies to endotoxin is useful in several medical colic diseases, including enteritis and peritonitis, or in any disease where loss of protein may be massive. Fresh plasma can also provide coagulation factors, fibronectin and immunoglobulins felt to be important in the defence against endotoxin. Plasma administration is indicated when the total plasma protein is below 4.0 g/dl. A minimum of 10 l is required to elevate the plasma protein level adequately in the adult horse, particularly when protein loss may be continuing.

Non-steroidal anti-inflammatory drugs inhibit cyclo-oxygenase activity, and thereby help reduce the production of prostaglandins during endotoxaemia. The use of flunixin meglumine helps to reduce the horse's response to endotoxin by completely blocking the production of thromboxane and prostacyclin (Hardee *et al.*, 1986; Moore *et al.*, 1986). Colic, diarrhoea, fever and pulmonary hypertension are all prevented when flunixin is administered during a sub-lethal challenge of endotoxin. Unfortunately, flunixin can mask the signs of impending shock without preventing fatal irreversible shock. Combined with fluid therapy, the use of flunixin is one of the most helpful treatments available for endotoxaemia, and its use is associated with an increased survival rate. Quarter to half the recommended dosage (0.125–0.25 mg/kg) can effectively shut down thromboxane and prostacyclin production and protect against the reaction to endotoxin release for 8 hours. This dosage may not be high enough to prevent pain from intestinal distension or mesenteric tension. Phenylbutazone does not provide the same protection from endotoxaemia as flunixin meglumine. Ketoprofen will provide protection similar to flunixin, and also blocks leukotriene production (Jackman *et al.*, 1994). Its usefulness in clinical cases is still not fully known.

Dopamine has been shown to help maintain the cardiovascular system during endotoxaemia, though it has been used most often during anaesthesia (Trim, 1982). It can be used at a dosage of 2.5–5.0 µg/kg per min as an intravenous drip. Its administration should be monitored using an ECG, as arrhythmias can occur. Intestinal motility can be inhibited during dopamine administration. Though it has not been used frequently in the conscious horse, it can have beneficial effects during the critical period when endotoxaemia is causing cardiovascular failure.

Before information about the equine systemic response to endo-toxaemia became available, corticosteroids were considered to be the treatment of choice for shock associated with colic. Corticosteroids have beneficial effects in hypovolaemic shock and septic shock in animals and humans. Even though the inhibitory effect of corticosteroids on phospholipase activity and tumour necrosis factor should prevent the initiation of the arachidonic acid transformation to prostaglandins, the protective effects in the horse with endotoxaemia are not as pronounced as with NSAIDs. To have a beneficial effect, corticosteroids must be given prior to endotoxin entering the system, making it almost impossible to use in a clinical situation. The possible potentiation of laminitis or a detrimental effect on healing is also a concern. Therefore, corticosteroids are not advocated in the treatment of endotoxaemia. If they are used, a sufficient dose should be given as a bolus prior to endotoxaemia, if it can be anticipated, or as soon as it is recognized. Dexamethasone dosage is 0.5–2 mg/kg.

Treatment of endotoxaemia with heparin is controversial. It is useful in preventing microthrombi and promoting anticoagulant activity of antithrombin III. Low-dose heparin (40 units/kg subcutaneously tid) has been used to help prevent signs of endotoxaemia and as a preventative for laminitis. In cases of impending disseminated intravascular coagulation (DIC), 100 units/kg tid intravenously are needed to provide anticoagulation. RBC aggregates have been found during treatment with heparin, increasing concern about plugging of capillaries. Presently, there is no specific recommendation for treatment for endotoxaemia unless a consumptive coagulopathy is predicted or diagnosed (White, 1990a).

One of the complicating factors associated with bowel ischaemia is the 'reperfusion injury'. This phenomenon can cause damage to the intestinal mucosa and serosa once reperfusion of an affected segment has occurred, or as the result of increased perfusion of organs after low flow or poor perfusion during shock. Reperfusion injury is caused by the release of toxic oxygen and hydroxyl radicals in the tissue, and by white blood cells, which have been attracted to injured tissue. The damage induced by these substances can cause continued endotoxin absorption due to the damaged intestinal mucosal barrier. Dimethyl sulphoxide (DMSO) is a hydroxyl radical scavenger, which has been used to reduce the injury normally observed during reperfusion. There are still questions concerning how effective DMSO is in sparing the mucosa from reperfusion injury in the horse, and there is limited proof that it is clinically beneficial to the horse during endotoxaemia (White, 1990a). Recently, intestinal permeability increases due to reperfusion were partially controlled with DMSO administration at a dose of 20 mg/kg. There have not been any apparent detrimental effects associated with its use clinically. DMSO also should be given as early as possible when shock is anticipated, or as soon as it is detected and the possibility for reperfusion exists. Clinical use is directed at preventing continuing intestinal injury, intestinal adhesions or laminar injury in the foot.

Modulation of intestinal motility

Ileus can be caused by numerous changes in the intestine. Known as paralytic ileus or adynamic ileus, the bowel has no physical obstruction but, rather, there is a lack of progressive motility. Stasis allows distension, which causes ischaemia of the wall and initiates fluid secretion into the bowel lumen. The cause may be reflex nervous inhibition due to sympathetic stimulation (alpha-receptor stimulation), local reduction of neurotransmitters in the myenteric plexuses, release of inhibitory neurotransmitters, or membrane damage from ischaemia, distension or inflammation affecting the function of nerves or muscle. Generally, the small intestine is the most susceptible to ileus. The caecum and large colon will frequently respond to laxative or cathartic therapy, and will not have long-term ileus after distension or impaction, or even after manipulation at surgery. The small intestine, on the other hand, may have ileus for long periods, resulting in accumulation of fluid in the stomach.

Stimulating intestinal motility and transit is usually not successful in the horse with severe intestinal disease. Once the intestine becomes ischaemic, oedematous or inflamed, the bowel is refractory to stimulation. The drugs commonly used are parasympathomimetic drugs (bethanecol), anticholinesterase drugs (neostigmine) or alpha-adrenergic blockers (phenoxybenzamine, acetylpromazine) (Adams, 1988). Cisapride directly stimulates the nerve of the cholinergic receptor, causing increased release of acetylcholine. All the nerve stimulating drugs, or drugs with direct cholinergic effect, are termed prokinetic drugs (Gerring, 1989). These drugs function in healthy intestine, which is able to react to stimuli. Other methods of gastrointestinal stimulation include exercise, and reducing intestinal distension by decompression. These simple methods are sometimes the most useful. Similarly, feeding will cause an increase in motility by volume loading and by intestinal reflex if the bowel is healthy. Allowing ingestion of food must be done with caution so as not to overload intestine which is already compromised and distended.

Direct or indirect stimulation can be beneficial in some instances. Metoclopramide appears to have some direct cholinergic activity and dopaminergic antagonism. It appears to have a beneficial effect on stomach emptying and small intestinal motility when used as a constant infusion at a rate of 0.1–0.5 mg/kg per hour (Adams, 1988). The lower dose has been used as a constant drip over several hours, or constantly until some response is seen. The higher doses can give more assured success but may cause untoward nervous signs, including ataxia, depression and excitement. Since individual horses have varying tolerance to the metoclopramide, titration is used to establish an effect. A recent report suggests administering metoclopramide continuously until a benefit is seen.

Bethanecol has also been useful in stimulating gastric emptying in cases of gastric ulceration when used at a dosage of 0.1–0.4 mg/kg *per os* or at a rate of approximately 0.01 mg/kg subcutaneously (White, 1990b). Neostigmine, an acetylcholinesterase inhibitor, can help stimulate propulsive motility of the colons, but it should not be used to treat impactions until the obstructing mass is soft enough to be easily moved. Though it produces some small intestinal activity, it decreases the propulsive activity of the jejunum and reduces normal gastric emptying. It is normally administered at 1–2 mg subcutaneously every 30–60 minutes to effect (White, 1990b). This has been recommended during and after surgery for small intestinal disease, but has little benefit over waiting for normal motility to return after the intestinal inflammation has been reduced. If pain is observed after neostigmine administration, it should be discontinued. This drug should not be used routinely for stimulation of motility; rather, it should be used as the last resort in stimulating motility for large intestinal ileus.

Erythromycin, another direct or prokinetic drug, is felt to increase motilin concentrations or act directly on motilin receptors, thereby increasing intestinal motility (Catnach and Fairclough, 1992). It is considered to work throughout the intestinal tract, but is most effective in the duodenum and has been shown to be effective in the caecum and colon of the horse for promoting progressive motility (Masri *et al.*, 1991). The dosage is 1 mg/kg intravenously. The drug may be useful for small intestinal disease, caecal impaction or other motility disorders. Though adverse reactions are not reported, diarrhoea in adult horses administered higher doses of erythromycin have been observed.

Alpha-adrenergic blockade has also been used with some success for small intestinal ileus. Acetylpromazine 0.01 mg/kg given every 4–6 hours has, in the author's experience, been effective in some horses with post-surgical small intestine ileus (White, 1990b). It should be used only after systemic hydration has returned to normal and when progressive colonic motility is evident but small intestinal activity is not yet sufficient to stop gastric reflux. Phenoxybenzamine, an alpha blocker similar to acetylpromazine, was clinically successful in reducing the duration of ileus (Beadle *et al.*, 1986). In these cases, it appears to reduce small intestinal reflux. Care should be taken when using this type of drug that the horse is monitored for capillary perfusion, as vasodilation can cause a dramatic drop in blood pressure.

Yohimbine has been shown to reverse ileus caused by endotoxin. This suggests that endotoxin stimulates alpha-adrenoreceptors in the bowel. The dosage is 0.15 mg/kg administered intravenously (Gerring and Hunt, 1986). It has not gained popularity in treating ileus, as it was not successful in an ileus model. Further work is indicated to ensure a proper dose is being used.

Flunixin meglumine and phenylbutazone inhibit production of prostaglandins. Prostaglandin production stimulated by endotoxaemia can reduce intestinal motility. The specific mechanism regarding ileus appears to be related to excessive production of PGE_2. Phenylbutazone 0.5–1.1 mg/kg appears to be more efficacious in maintaining motility compared to flunixin meglumine, but both appear to help in treating ileus (King and Gerring, 1989). These compounds have a prostaglandin-independent effect on motility similar to yohimbine. Acting as alpha-adrenergic blockers, they can help reduce the ileus due to sympathetic stimulation.

Several treatments with unknown mechanisms have been tried in horses, but their success is not yet determined. Lidocaine administration has recently been investigated as a way to treat ileus (Malone and Turner, 1994). Administered as a 1.3 mg/kg bolus and continued as a constant infusion of 0.05 mg/kg per min intravenously, it produces blood levels of 1–2 mg/l. The mechanism of action is not known, though administration significantly decreases postoperative pain. It has been speculated that it blocks nerve endings, thereby blocking sympathetic stimulation. It must be used carefully. Side effects, include bradycardia, muscle fasciculations progressing to ataxia and eventually recumbency, were associated with blood levels of 2.4–2.6 mg/l. All signs resolve upon decreasing the administration rate.

Calcium administration can help induce intestinal contractions, particularly if there is a serum calcium deficit. It is normally administered as a drip with other intravenous fluids. A total dose of 50–100 g is normally sufficient until calcium levels can be measured to assure adequate concentrations are present. Calcium administration is particularly useful in colon distension and atony, and should be considered in postpartum mares with below normal calcium levels during colic. Supplementation of calcium in intravenous fluid is possible, but caution is advised because administration of these solutions too rapidly may cause cardiac arrhythmias.

Hypomagnesaemia can also cause ileus. This is particularly true in horses with ileus that have been off feed for some time. Serum magnesium should be monitored along with other electrolytes, particularly in cases with prolonged ileus. When magnesium is low, it commonly requires long-term supplementation until the horse is back on a normal diet. Cardiac arrhythmias are also possible with low magnesium concentrations, and may be the first indication that such a problem is present.

Lubricants or laxatives can help to soften food impactions or remove sand impactions. Mineral oil helps to coat the intestinal tract and softens the contents. The more emulsified the oil, the greater its ability to penetrate ingesta and the more likely that the oil can be absorbed by the intestine. Although reported to coat the intestinal tract and block the absorption of toxins, there is no documentation of these statements. Its use is well established for impaction colic, and it is indicated whenever a case of impaction in the large colon or small colon is diagnosed. The dosage is normally 5–10 ml/kg (half to one gallon) of mineral oil for a 450 kg horse.

Mineral oil can serve as a fluid marker to determine the transit time of fluids through the tract. Normally it will be recognized in the faeces as an oily coating within 12–18 hours. Seeing mineral oil in faeces or at the anus does not always mean that an impaction has cleared, since the oil can move around the mass and not penetrate the impaction. This is particularly true with sand or foreign body impaction. Mineral oil should not therefore be considered the only alternative for treating an impaction or other forms of mild colic.

Mineral oil can be misused for treating colic. Almost all horses with colic have mineral oil administered as a matter of tradition. However, it should never be given to a horse suspected of having any form of strangulation obstruction or to a horse with severe pain where the diagnosis cannot be made. In these cases it can complicate the problem. In the case of small intestinal obstruction, dosing with mineral oil can increase the volume of sequestered fluid and therefore the stomach dilatation.

Ionic cathartics can soften the mass by increasing the intraluminal water content of the intestine or inducing reflex propulsive motility. This increase in water will overload the colon with water and decrease the transit time. Magnesium sulphate (Epsom salts) is a potent cathartic that can be used to hydrate faeces and to help flush sand from the colon. The dosage is 500 g/day for 3 days, repeated after 7 days. Magnesium sulphate appears to cause a reflex secretion of fluid into the intestinal tract, particularly in the colon and small colon. Its action is immediate, and the actual benefit from an osmotic effect may not be as great as once thought.

The docusates (dioctyl sodium sulphosuccinate) (DSS) are surface-active agents, which increase the secretion from the intestinal mucosa. They can cause irritation and toxicity at high dosages. Normally a 10 per cent solution of DSS is used, administering 10–30 mg/kg via stomach tube. Doubling this dose or using DSS for more than 3 days may cause dehydration and bowel irritation. This cathartic is effective in breaking up impactions partly due to the surfactant effect, which can help water penetrate firm masses of ingesta. Other stimulants such as cascara sagrada and danthron are very irritating, and should not be used in the horse with an intestinal disturbance.

Bulk-forming laxatives made of cellulose derivatives, such as psyllium, methylcellulose and carboxymethycellulose, can be used in the horse. These are used for the treatment of ingested sand and sand impaction, and have recently been used to help resolve caecal impactions. They do not have a rapid cathartic effect, and need to be used over several days for a laxative effect. The mechanism of action is hydrophilic; by increasing the water content in the bowel lumen it speeds up bowel evacuation, and at the same time evacuation of sand with the water. The dosage is approximately 1 g/kg in about 2 l of water once or twice daily, usually for 2–3 days. These cathartics have no disadvantages except for clogging stomach pumps and tubes, as the mixtures tend to gel quickly when mixed with water. They should not be relied upon to clear impactions of ingesta, as their laxative effect can take days to occur. Even when used for days, there may not be a marked softening of the faeces despite an increase in the water content.

A balanced electrolyte solution administered intravenously will sometimes provide a stimulus for intestinal motility. This has been recognized as a response to hydration and correction of electrolyte imbalances, and addition of volume to the intestine due to secretion. This treatment works particularly well for colon impaction, and appears to stimulate motility in cases of ileus of the caecum and large colon. 'Overhydration' with lactated Ringer's solution or acetated Ringer's solution at 40–80 l every 24 hours helps to provide adequate secretion of fluid to soften hardened impactions.

Feeding

The horse with gastrointestinal disorders needs to have a source of nutrition as soon as possible in order to maintain a positive energy balance. There is no information regarding the degree of insult to fermentation and the production of volatile fatty acids that occurs after colic, intestinal surgery or instances of intestinal emptying or lavage. Most horses appear to respond rapidly, with weight gain and normal intestinal transit, once feeding is started. The feeding schedule is determined by the disease encountered and the degree of ileus.

With small intestinal disease, the horse is held off all food and water until:

1. There is no more gastric reflux.
2. The horse has stopped sequestering fluid in the small bowel as indicated by a rectal examination, and balancing of hydration on maintenance levels of fluids has been achieved.
3. The sounds of the caecum have become progressive and characteristically fluid, indicating the successful transit of fluid from the small intestine into the caecum.

Other signs, including an intense desire by the horse to drink, should be ignored until these basic criteria can be met.

After the intestine is known to be functioning, water is offered to horses at about 1 l (approximately six swallows at 150 ml per swallow) every 30–60 minutes until there is assurance that there is no further sequestration by the bowel or stomach. Once oral water can be tolerated, it is made available at all times. If this is successful for 24 hours, feeding of hay can be initiated, again in small amounts, given every 2–3 hours. It is best to measure the amount of hay at 0.25–0.5 kg. Any type of hay appears appropriate, but only one type should be used until normal faecal transit has been established. Alfalfa hay often has a laxative effect, and can serve as the sole source of feed until intestinal transit is re-established. As soon as the horse can tolerate a full diet, the hay should be made available at all times.

With diseases of the colon or caecum, water can often be offered immediately unless the horse has no intestinal sounds, in which case intravenous fluid is relied upon for hydration. Hay is fed as soon as possible to help stimulate motility. However, this is offered in small amounts every 1–4 hours while monitoring to assure that borborygmi are still present and that transit of ingesta is commencing or returning to normal. Monitoring of the rectal findings in horses with a caecal or large colon impaction should be carried out, and no feed given until the impaction is no longer palpable and there is evidence of transit of ingesta through the intestine. Return to a full hay diet is gradual until normal transit of ingesta is established. Horses after surgery for large colon or caecal disease should be held off feed for at least 12 hours, or until there is evidence of intestinal transit. Small colon disease may require a reduction in the amount of ingesta being passed. Horses with resection and anastomosis of the small colon are fed a low volume diet of alfalfa pellets or a total horse ration for about 10 days before starting hay. Similarly, horses with adhesions or intestinal lesions that could lead to stenosis are fed small amounts of a total pelleted diet to avoid bulk and large fibre intake.

The resumption of feeding grain should only occur after the horse has normal transit of feed for 1 week. The grain fed should be increased in amount, gradually bringing the horse back to the pre-colic level or preferred level over a 5–7 day period. Often it is wise to review the diet to see if the total amount of grain being fed should be reduced permanently. Though the energy requirement of horses with an acute abdomen are no doubt increased, a slow increase in the energy delivered orally is appropriate until transit of ingesta is considered normal. This area requires further research, to establish the best method to maintain adequate energy intake.

In some cases oral nutrition is not possible, and parenteral nutrition can be used to supply part or all of the horse's energy needs for several days or weeks. A horse requires 18 kcal/kg for basal maintenance at absolute rest, and up to 35 kcal/kg for maintenance. This quantity may be substantially higher in horses with intestinal disease or infection. The basal requirement of approximately 18 kcal/kg can be used as the goal for partial parenteral nutrition. Parenteral nutrients include glucose, amino acids and lipids. Glucose supplies approximately 4 kcal/g, while lipids can deliver almost twice that amount. When calculating the amount of each nutrient to use, the total caloric needs are considered. In cases of short-term energy supplementation, partial parenteral nutrition is considered adequate and, in this situation, glucose is used as the chief energy source. A 500 kg horse will require 500×18 kcal = 9000 kcal per day. Dividing 9000 by 4 kcal/g gives 2250 g of glucose, or 4500 ml of 50 per cent glucose. The horse will also require approximately 1 g nitrogen (grams of protein/6.25 = grams of nitrogen) per 200 kcal. For partial parenteral nutrition, therefore, 45 g nitrogen or about 300 g protein or amino acids are needed in the solution. Most amino acid solutions are 8.5–10 per cent solutions; therefore, 3 l of 10 per cent amino acid solution and 4500 ml of 50 per cent dextrose are mixed and administered by intravenous catheter over an 18–24 hour period to supplement the energy needs of the horse. Initially half this amount is administered, to prevent hyperglycaemia with glucosuria. A 48-hour break between periods is usually sufficient to prevent intolerance to the glucose. In cases where full parenteral nutrition is felt to be required, 10 per cent solutions of lipids are recommended to make up 30–60 per cent of the energy source. Lipids deliver higher energy (9 kcal/g) and are isotonic, which reduces the irritation that can be seen when using glucose as the total energy source. Horses may be less tolerant of lipids if endotoxaemia is present but, in most clinical situations, lipids are accepted better than the high levels of glucose. Parenteral nutrition can be beneficial in maintaining protein levels, and can maintain the positive energy balance needed for healing and intestinal function. This therapy should be considered immediately if ileus, shock, or peritonitis do not allow oral alimentation.

References

Adams, R. and McClure, J. J. (1985). Acute renal dysfunction: A review of 38 equine cases and discussion of diagnostic parameters. *Proc. Am. Assoc. Equine Pract., Ann. Conv.*, 635–47.

Adams, S. B. (1988). Recognition and management of ileus. *Vet. Clin. N. Am. Equine Pract.*, **4**, 91–104.

Adams, S. B., Lamar, C. H. and Masty, J. (1984). Motility of the distal portion of the jejunum and pelvic flexure in ponies: effects of six drugs. *Am. J. Vet. Res.*, **45**, 795–9.

Beadle, R. E., Brooks, D. E. and Martin, G. S. (1986). Phenoxybenzamine as an adjunct in the therapy for ileus in the horse. In *Equine Colic Research Symposium* (T. D. Byars and N. A. White, eds), pp. 112–15. University of Georgia.

Catnach, S. M. and Fairclough, P. D. G. (1992). Erythromycin and the gut. *Gut*, **33**, 379–401.

Clark, E. S. and Moore, J. N. (1989). The effects of slow infusion of a low dosage of endotoxin in healthy horses. *Equine Vet. J.*, **7**, 33–7.

Dabareiner, D. M. and White, N. A. (1995). Large colon impaction in horses: 147 cases (1985–1991). *J. Am. Vet. Med. Assoc.*, **206**, 679–85.

Davies, J. V. and Gerring, E. L. (1983). Effect of spasmolytic analgesic drugs on the motility patterns of the equine small intestine. *Res. Vet. Sci.*, **34**, 334–9.

Ducharme, N. G. and Fubini, S. L. (1983). Gastrointestinal complications associated with the use of atropine in horses. *J. Am. Vet. Med. Assoc.*, **182**, 229–31.

Garner, H. E., Sprouse, R. F. and Green, E. M. (1985). Active and passive immunization for blockage of endotoxemia. *Proc. Am. Assoc. Equine. Pract. Ann. Conv.*, pp. 525–32.

Gerring, E. L. (1989). Effects of pharmacological agents on gastrointestinal motility. *Vet. Clin. N. Am. Equine Pract.*, **5**, 283–94.

Gerring, E. E. L. and Hunt, J. M. (1986). Pathophysiology of equine post-operative ileus: effect of adrenergic blockade, parasympathetic stimulation and metoclopramide in an experimental model. *Equine Vet. J.*, **18**, 249–55.

Hardee, M. M., Moore, J. N. and Hardee, G. E. (1986). Effects of flunixin meglumine, phenylbutazone and a selective thromboxane synthetase inhibitor

(UK-38 485) on thromboxane and prostacyclin production in healthy horses. *Res. Vet. Sci.*, **40**, 152–6.

Jackman, B. R., Moore, J. N., Barton, M. H. and Morris, D. D. (1994). Comparison of the effects of ketoprofen and flunixin meglumine on the *in vitro* response of equine peripheral blood monocytes to bacterial endotoxin. *Can. J. Vet. Res.*, **58**, 138–43.

Kalpravidh, M. (1984). Analgesics for equine colic: a literature review and clinical experience. *Thai J. Vet. Med.*, **14**, 241–50.

King, J. N. and Gerring, E. L. (1989). Antagonism of endotoxin-induced disruption of equine bowel motility by flunixin and phenylbutazone. *Equine Vet. J.*, **7**, 38–42.

Lowe, J. E. (1978). Xylazine, pentazocine, meperidine, and dipyrone for relief of balloon-induced equine colic: a double-blind comparative evaluation. *J. Equine Med. Surg.*, **3**, 286–91.

Lowe, J. E. and Hilfiger, J. (1984). Analgesic and sedative effects of detomidine in a colic model: blind studies on efficacy and duration of effects. *Proc. Am. Assoc. Equine Pract.*, **30**, 225–34.

Lowe, J. E. and Hilfiger, J. (1986). Analgesic and sedative effects of detomidine compared to xylazine in a colic model using i.v. and i.m. routes of administration. *Acta Vet. Scand.*, **82**, 85–95.

Lowe, J. E., Sellers, A. F. and Brondum, J. (1980). Equine pelvic flexure impaction. A model used to evaluate motor events and compare drug response. *Cornell Vet.*, **70**, 401–12.

MacKay, R. J. (1992). Endotoxaemia. In *Current Therapy in Equine Medicine* (N. Robinson, ed.),pp. 225–32. W. B. Saunders.

Malone, E. D. and Turner, E. D. (1994). Intravenous lidocaine for the treatment of ileus in the horse. *5th Equine Colic Research Symposium, Athens, Georgia*, p. 39. University of Georgia.

Masri, M. D., Merritt, A. M. and Burrow, J. A. (1991). Effect of erythromycin on equine colonic motility. *4th Equine Colic Research Symposium, Athens, Georgia*, p. 47. University of Georgia.

Moore, J. N. (1985). Management of pain and shock in equine colic. *Comp. Cont. Ed. Pract. Vet.*, **7**, S169–73.

Moore, J. N. (1990). Pathophysiology of circulatory shock. In *The Equine Acute Abdomen* (N. A. White, ed.), pp. 90–99. Lea and Febiger.

Moore, J. N., Garner, H. E., Shapland, J. E. and Schaub, R. G. (1981). Equine endotoxaemia: an insight into cause and treatment. *J. Am. Vet. Med. Assoc.*, **179**, 473–7.

Moore, J. N., Hardee, M. M. and Hardee, G. E. (1986). Modulation of arachidonic acid metabolism in endotoxic horses: Comparison of flunixin meglumine, pheylbutazone, and a selective thromboxane synthetase inhibitor. *Am. J. Vet. Res.*, **47**, 110–13.

Muir, W. W. and Robertson, J. T. (1985). Visceral analgesia: effects of xylazine, butorphanol, meperidine and pentazocine in horses. *Am. J. Vet. Res.*, **46**, 2081–4.

Muir, W. W., Robertson, J. T., Wade, A. and Grospitch, B. (1982). Pharmacological effects of intravenous butorphanol tartrate in horses. *Proc. Equine Colic Res. Symp., September*, pp. 223–4.

Pippi, N. L. and Lumb, W. V. (1979). Objective tests of analgesic drugs in ponies. *Am. J. Vet. Res.*, **40**, 1082–6.

Robertson, J. R., Muir, W. W. and Sams, R. (1981). Cariopulmonary effects of butorphanol tartrate in horses. *Am. J. Vet. Res.*, **41**, 2474–9.

Semrad, S. D., Hardee, G. E., Hardee, M. M. and Moore, J. N. (1985). Flunixin meglumine give in small doses: Pharmacokinetics and prostaglandin inhibition in healthy horses. *Am. J. Vet. Res.*, **46**, 2474–9.

Sojka, J. E., Adams, S. B., Lamar, C. H. and Eller, L. L. (1988). Effect of butorphanol, pentazocine, meperidine or metoclopramide on intestinal motility in female ponies. *Am. J. Vet. Res.*, **49**, 527–9.

Spier, S. J., Lavoie, J. P., Cullor, J. S. *et al.* (1989). Protection against clinical endotoxaemia in horses by using plasma containing antibody ato a Rc mutant *E. coli* (J5). *Circ. Shock*, **28,** 235.

Trim, C. M. (1982). Investigation of the cardiovascular effects of dopamine infusion in anaesthetized horses. *Proc. Equine Colic Res. Symp., September*, pp. 227–31.

Virtanen, R. (1986). Pharmacology of detomidine and other alpha2-adrenoceptor agonists in the brain. *Acta Vet. Scand.*, **82,** 36–46.

White, N. A. (1990a). Intensive care, monitoring, and complications of acute abdominal disease. In *The Equine Acute Abdomen* (N. A. White, ed.), pp. 310–35. Lea and Febiger.

White, N. A. (1990b). Treatment to alter intestinal motility. In *The Equine Acute Abdomen* (N. A. White, ed.), pp. 178–84. Lea and Febiger.

White, N. A. (1992). Fluid therapy in the horse. In *Veterinary Gastroenterology* (N. V. Anderson, ed.), 2nd edn, pp. 119–29. Lea and Febiger.

4

Management of specific diseases

Ileus/spasmodic colic

Simple colic, one of the most frequent types of colic, is the least understood. Often this problem is related to stasis of bowel apparently causing a functional obstruction, or a spasm of the bowel resulting in pain. There is no one cause, and frequently these episodes go unexplained. This type of colic makes up more than 80 per cent of the colic observed in a normal population. Parasites are blamed for many of these colic episodes.

Clinical signs

Signs of simple colic include mild to moderate pain, frequently intermittent, which is easily controlled with analgesics. Lack of intestinal sounds leads to a diagnosis of ileus, whereas increased borborygmi indicate a spasmodic colic. Though the heart rate may be slightly elevated, most of the vital signs are normal. Tympany or flatulence, also called gas colic, may be indicated by auscultation or by palpation *per rectum*. Often, pain is the only sign and may be mild.

Treatment

Treatment for the functional obstructions is symptomatic. Analgesics such as non-steroidal anti-inflammatory drugs (flunixin meglumine) or alpha agonists (xylazine or detomidine) are usually curative. Traditionally, most horses are treated with mineral oil as a lubricant. Some horses respond to walking, or the pain may resolve with time. The common treatments for these problems are described in Chapter 3, *Medical Treatments*.

Treatment of gas accumulation in the large colon or caecum (also called gas colic) usually only involves analgesics to allow the gas to pass through the intestinal tract. In some cases decompression may be necessary, either by percutaneous aspiration of the caecum or by abdominal surgery.

Small intestine

The small intestine of the horse is prone to mechanical obstruction from a wide variety of causes (Table 4.1). The obstruction may be simple or, more frequently, strangulating in nature. These diseases are characterized by fluid sequestration in the small intestine and stomach. The resulting signs include gastric reflux, dehydration and distended small intestines.

Table 4.1 Small intestine obstruction

Simple obstruction	Intraluminal	Feed impaction
		Ascarids
		Foreign body
	Intramural	Neoplasia
		Muscular hypertrophy
	Compression	Adhesions
		Abscessation
		Fibrous bands
		Non-strangulating pedunculated lipoma
Strangulation obstruction	Hernias	External (umbilical, inguinal/ scrotal, ventral)
		Internal (epiploic foramen, diaphragmatic, mesenteric, various ligaments)
	Intussusception	Jejuno-jejunal
		Ileo-ileal
		Ileocaecal
	Volvulus	

Simple obstruction

Impaction with dry ingesta (or, much less frequently, with ascarid worms) is the most common cause of complete simple obstruction of the small intestine. The ileum with its narrow lumen and muscular wall is the most common site.

The aetiology is uncertain, but feed with a high fibre content has been implicated as a major cause. The incidence is particularly high in the Southern United States, where Coastal Bermuda grass hay is commonly fed (Embertson, 1985). Ileal muscular hypertrophy has been reported as a common finding (Allen, 1985) but, in the author's experience, the majority of obstructions in the UK are primary impactions with no evidence of ileal or ileocaecal orifice pathology. Ileal impaction is not infrequently found at laparotomy or autopsy in cases of acute grass sickness.

Clinical signs

The condition is characterized by sudden onset, moderate to severe abdominal pain, which often subsides in 6–10 hours before recurring as secondary gastric distension develops. Distended loops of fluid-filled small intestine can be felt on rectal examination in the caudal abdomen. Early on in the course of the condition, a firm, unyielding impaction measuring 40–100 cm or more in length may be felt to the left of the base of the caecum. Progressive sequestration of fluid in the more proximal small intestine and, eventually, the stomach occurs over 24 hours. The packed cell volume and total plasma protein rise progressively, and there is a concurrent rise in heart rate as hypovolaemia develops. Serum electrolyte concentrations are generally normal and as hypovolaemia becomes evident, most horses have a moderate metabolic acidosis.

Abdominal auscultation reveals decreased or absent intestinal sounds. Peritoneal fluid remains normal in appearance until the obstruction has been in existence 20 hours or more, when an increase in total protein and leucocyte count occurs in response to ischaemia of the distended intestine.

Treatment

Although medical therapy (including analgesics, spasmolytics, intravenous fluid therapy and mineral oil by nasogastric tube) has been recommended, conservative treatment is usually unsuccessful unless the impaction is relatively soft and involves only a very short length of ileum. If serial rectal palpations show persistent, more extensive small intestinal distension rather than a progressively smaller, softer impaction, continued medical therapy is not justified and prompt surgical intervention is indicated.

The impacted ileum, which is readily identified via a ventral midline coeliotomy, can be cleared by gently breaking down the dehydrated ingesta by pressure applied to the intestinal wall and then manually massaging it in an oral direction into the fluid contents of 1–2 m distal jejunum, which have been withdrawn from the abdomen. Once the ingesta has been put into suspension, it can be stripped into the caecum. If this method proves difficult, saline injected into the mass of ingesta will aid its dispersal. A note should be made of any resistance to the passage of the suspended ingesta through the distal ileum and the ileocaecal orifice, which should be checked for hypertrophy of the ileal wall or a doughnut-like thickening of the caecal mucosa at the orifice. These are sometimes encountered in horses with heavy tapeworm infestations. If there is any suspicion of distal ileal hypertrophy, the risk of re-impaction can be avoided by carrying out a side-to-side anastomosis between proximal ileum and caecum (Embertson, 1985). However, the author has found this to be necessary in no more than 5 per cent of cases.

The prognosis in ileal impaction is largely related to the duration of colic before surgery. Reported survival rates have varied from 47 per cent (White, 1985) to 86.3 per cent (Huskamp, 1982).

Ascarid impaction can occur in young foals and yearlings with heavy burdens of *Parascaris equorum*, and usually follows the administration of an effective anthelmintic. Although in some cases the obstruction is temporary, in others enterotomy is necessary to evacuate the gut of the large number of dead worms.

Foreign body obstruction is rare in horses.

Ileal hypertrophy

Hypertrophy of the muscular layers of the distal ileum brings about progressive obstruction resulting in intermittent colic, which becomes more frequent and severe as the obstruction develops. The aetiology is uncertain, but neurogenic stenosis and stenosis following strongyle larval migration have been suggested as possible causes. However, there is increasing evidence that heavy infestation with the tapeworm *Anaplocephala perfoliata* causes similar changes.

Over a period of a few weeks, several metres of terminal jejunum become dilated and thick-walled in response to the slowly developing occlusive lesion. Palpation of this hypertrophied jejunum on rectal examination indicates a chronic obstruction. In most cases, the obstruction can be successfully bypassed with a side-to-side ileocaecal anastomosis without the need to resect any bowel. If tapeworm involvement is suspected, the horse is treated with pyrantel pamoate at 38 mg/kg body weight.

Neoplasia

Neoplasia is an uncommon cause of obstruction in the horse. Lymphosarcoma is the most common neoplasm, and may present as a single primary lesion or as extensive lesions, usually involving the mesenteric lymph nodes. Clinical signs include weight loss, variable appetite and low-grade abdominal pain over a period of several weeks. The mass itself, together with hypertrophied jejunum proximal to the obstruction, can be recognized *per rectum*.

Euthanasia is necessary when secondary lesions are present in the lymph nodes, but horses with single localized lesions can recover following resection of the affected portion of the gut and an anastomosis.

Fibrous bands

Obstruction by fibrous bands may vary from localized stricture to strangulation of several metres of intestine. The exact nature and cause of the bands can be difficult to determine. In many cases they have to be cut blindly, deep within the abdomen, thus precluding close scrutiny. Some appear to be attached to mesentery, others to the intestine, viscera or the abdominal wall. In young animals they may be congenital in origin.

Adhesions

Adhesions between peritoneal surfaces may be a sequel to peritonitis or previous abdominal surgery, particularly small intestine resection. Adhesions produce kinking or compression of bowel, or may predispose to volvulus or internal herniation. Obstruction by a solitary band of adhesion can be removed by sectioning but, due to the marked tendency for adhesions to recur when they are more extensive, the obstruction may be managed by bypassing the intestine involved, or euthanasia may be considered the appropriate course of action.

Abdominal abscess

The majority of internal abdominal abscesses found in the mesenteric lymph nodes are believed to be the result of systemic spread of respiratory infections. Others may be a sequel to foreign body penetration or umbilical infection. As the abscess enlarges and the associated adhesive peritonitis becomes more extensive, the adjacent small intestine is compressed and constricted. Intermittent colic and chronic weight loss over a period of several weeks are common clinical signs, although a large abdominal abscess can go unsuspected until the horse develops acute, complete obstruction. Rectal examination may provide an indication whether or not surgery is likely to be successful. A localized, well-encapsulated, mobile mesenteric abscess may be revealed. More often, however, the abscess is very large, involves loops of bowel and is firmly attached deep within the abdomen, thus preventing exteriorization. In these cases, surgery to free, resect or bypass the obstructed intestine often proves futile.

Strangulation obstruction

Strangulation obstruction may be due to external or internal hernias, pedunculated lipomas or small intestine volvulus.

External hernias

Umbilical hernia

Strangulation of intestine in an umbilical hernia is relatively rare. Incarceration, which quickly leads to strangulation, is characterized by acute onset of abdominal pain and a painful irreducible swelling at the umbilicus. The hernial sac is carefully incised under general anaesthetic to expose the entrapped intestine, which is freed by enlarging the defect in the abdominal wall. Any compromised intestine is resected. Even if the entrapped gut can be reduced by gentle pressure at the initial examination, it is often advisable to anaesthetize the foal and open the abdominal cavity in order to examine the small intestine for evidence of infarction. It is not uncommon to find a circular area of the ileal wall, which had been trapped in the constricting hernial ring, showing infarctive change. This could lead to perforation. This partial herniation of the side of a segment of intestine is known as a Richter's hernia, and can also involve a pouch of caecum.

Inguinal hernia

Acquired inguinal hernia or scrotal hernia in the stallion is usually indirect, unilateral, and almost always produces complete intestinal obstruction. Standard-bred horses have been reported to have a breed disposition to inguinal hernia, and warmblood, saddlebred and Tennessee walking horses appear to have the same tendency.

A sudden increase in intra-abdominal pressure during service, strenuous exercise or abdominal trauma may precede inguinal herniation and allow displacement of intestine by altering the anatomy of the inguinal canal.

The herniated jejunum or, more frequently, ileum passes through the vaginal ring into the cavity of the tunica vaginalis parietalis, and lies in direct contact with the spermatic cord and testis. Although the intestine passes through the vaginal ring, the site of incarceration is some 2–3 cm distal to it at the distal end of the funnel-shaped beginning of the vaginal process, where the internal spermatic fascia changes to loose connective tissue (Huskamp, 1998a). Incarcerated bowel becomes strangulated within 4–6 hours. This type of obstruction should always be suspected in a stallion presenting with colic. Examination of the scrotum may or may not show enlargement. Due to pressure exerted on the cord by the loop of intestine, which interferes with lymphatic and venous drainage, the affected testis is frequently enlarged and is cool and firm to the touch. The presence of distended small intestine palpable *per rectum* at the deep inguinal ring will confirm the diagnosis. Ultrasonography at the neck of the scrotum may also be used to demonstrate small intestine within the vaginal process.

In early cases, the intestine can be retracted from the inguinal ring by traction *per rectum*. Depending on the length of time the bowel has been trapped, it may cause obstruction or become infarcted. Most cases require immediate surgery. At surgery the hernia is best reduced by simult-aneous pressure applied to the loop of intestine, after opening into the vaginal sac, and traction applied to the intestine via a short midline incision. The constricting tissue frequently has to be cut carefully using Metzenbaum scissors, even if the obstructed loop is decompressed by suction. Resection of the herniated bowel *in situ* is not an option when, as is most frequently the case, it comprises ileum.

One surgeon (von Plocki, 1995) used a curved bistoury placed through the abdominal incision to cut the vaginal ring without incising the scrotum. Once the vaginal ring is enlarged, the herniated intestine is withdrawn into the abdomen from the ventral midline incision. In this instance, the testicle is preserved and the vaginal ring left to heal without suturing. In the cases reported, the affected testicle has not been a problem. Though not reported, a higher risk for recurrence must be considered when using this technique.

The released segment of gut is returned to the abdominal cavity, and the decision whether or not resection is necessary delayed until the testis has been removed and the inguinal canal obliterated by twisting the vaginal sac into a pedicle and ligating it with a transfixing ligature, which is anchored to the margin of the external inguinal ring. In many cases the bowel improves markedly after the strangulation has been released and, because short segments of intestine are usually involved, resection is not necessary (Freeman, 1997).

Salvage of the testis on the affected side is not usually an option because of its impaired viability. Whether the remaining testis should be removed is a matter of some debate, but owners should be appraised of the possible hereditary implications in the breeds mentioned above.

Congenital scrotal hernia in foals does not lead to incarceration and colic unless intestine passes through a tear in the common tunic, when the severe scrotal and preputial swelling and abdominal discomfort that follow are indications for immediate surgery.

Ventral hernia

Small intestine may herniate through breaches in the abdominal wall resulting from external trauma. Surprisingly, despite the 'grid-iron' nature of the defect there is often no vascular compromise to the herniated intestine and little or no compression of its lumen. If this is the case, surgery to return the intestine to the abdominal cavity and repair the defect in the abdominal wall is best delayed for 8–10 days to allow an increase in tensile strength of the damaged tissues.

Internal hernias

Small intestine may displace through a normal or pathological opening within the abdominal cavity, the consequence of which is usually a strangulating obstruction. Potential openings such as the epiploic foramen and nephrosplenic space, or pathological defects or tears of the mesentery, omentum and the various ligaments (which include the gastrosplenic, gastrohepatic and uterine broad ligaments) are sites of internal hernia.

Epiploic foramen

Incarceration of the small intestine through the epiploic foramen is one of the most common forms of internal hernia in the horse, and is especially common in the older animal. The epiploic foramen, the relatively narrow passage through which the greater and lesser omental sacs communicate, is situated on the visceral surface of the liver dorsal to the portal fissure. In older horses, as the right lobe of the liver atrophies, the foramen enlarges, thereby making it easier for a loop of small intestine to enter. However, the possibility of epiploic foramen incarceration should not be ignored in young horses. Thirty-nine per cent of cases seen by the author were in horses less than 7 years of age, and these included two yearlings.

The intestine may enter the foramen from right to left, or, much more frequently, left to right. Although jejunum alone may be involved, ileum is frequently incarcerated. The length of bowel involved can vary from as little as 10 cm to 17 m. Strangulation obstruction occurs in approximately 87 per cent of cases, while in the remainder, vascular impairment is minimal. In these horses with simple obstruction, a localized impaction is frequently found in the herniated loop.

There is usually sudden onset of abdominal pain which, when strangulation obstruction is present, is very severe and unresponsive to analgesic therapy. Though there is little to distinguish it from any other acute strangulation obstruction, a marked pain response to traction on the caudal band of the caecum during rectal examination and demonstration of small intestine in the right dorsal quadrant by ultrasonography are suggestive of this disease.

During exploratory surgery, palpation of small intestine other than the duodenum on its short mesentery in the right dorsal quadrant of the abdomen will confirm the diagnosis. The direction of the herniation can be determined by tracing small intestine orally from the ileocaecal junction to the epiploic foramen.

Reduction of the hernia is carried out by very gentle traction aided, if necessary, by suction and manual decompression of the obstructed loop. In order to avoid damage to the portal vein and resulting fatal haemorrhage, traction should be applied in the plane of the foramen and no attempt should be made to dilate or enlarge the foramen. Irreversibly damaged intestine is resected. When simple obstruction complicated by an impaction exists, dispersal of the impacted material prior to reduction of the hernia is facilitated by pulling a metre of fluid-filled intestine proximal to the obstruction through the foramen before breaking down the mass by digital pressure.

Recurrence of epiploic foramen incarceration several months or years later has been seen in a small number of cases.

Diaphragmatic hernia

Diaphragmatic defects may be congenital or acquired. Most follow thoracic or abdominal trauma or events that produce sudden increases in intra-abdominal pressure, such as strenuous exercise, parturition or extreme gastrointestinal distension.

If small intestine is displaced, signs of intestinal obstruction predominate, often with a rapidly fatal outcome. In some cases, virtually all the small intestine apart from the relatively fixed duodenum and ileum pass into the chest, and as a result the abdominal cavity appears and feels more empty than normal. Abdominocentesis usually reveals peritoneal fluid that is normal in colour; the sanguinous fluid normally associated with strangulation obstruction being present in large volumes in the thoracic cavity. Lateral radiographs of the chest will show partial obliteration of the normal caudal lung shadow by this fluid and the herniated intestine, but such investigations are not necessary to arrive at a decision to perform exploratory surgery. Ultrasonography may also help to visualize loops of distended small intestine in the thorax.

Horses with diaphragmatic hernias present a major challenge to anaesthetists, and may die on induction. Tears resulting from trauma are usually relatively large, and present no difficulty in identification. However, the author has encountered a number of cases where small intestine has passed through a small hole, presumed to be congenital. This has required enlarging the defect with scissors or a Roberts' guarded embryotomy knife before the strangulated gut, often several metres in length, can be removed from the chest. Most tears can be closed with difficulty by direct suture apposition of the edges or by the use of a mesh implant, but some inaccessible ones have to be left unsutured. If these are not subsequently occluded by adhesions, recurrence of herniation is likely. Stainless steel staples to attach a mesh to the defect may allow closure of defects in the dorsal regions of the diaphragm.

Mesenteric hernias

Most mesenteric hernias involve defects in the mesentery of the small intestine whilst others involve that of the large or small colon. Some mesenteric hernias are associated with congenital defects or remnants of the vitelline artery, a mesodiverticular band. The majority of defects are acquired as the result of trauma such as a violent blow to the abdomen or surgical manipulation of the bowel. A loop of small intestine passes through the tear and becomes incarcerated and strangulated. A volvulus of the incarcerated bowel frequently follows.

The clinical signs are consistent with a strangulating small intestinal obstruction. Prominent signs include pain, distended small intestine and gastric reflux once distension causes fluid retention in the stomach.

Treatment includes immediate surgery, with reduction of the hernia and correction of a volvulus if present. Enlargement of the hernial opening may be necessary. Resection of the strangulated bowel is performed, and if this has not included the defective mesentery every effort should be made to close the rent to avoid a recurrence of herniation.

However, a defect situated near the root of the mesentery can be extremely difficult to suture. Defects in the gastrosplenic ligament, meso-duodenum and broad ligament are impossible to close.

Intussusceptions

Intussusceptions in the horse most commonly involve the small intestine. Most involve ileum, with jejunal intussusceptions being much less common.

Ileal intussusceptions are seen particularly in young horses. They may involve invagination of a few centimetres of terminal ileum into itself, forming a doughnut-like ring close to the ileocaecal junction, or varying lengths of ileum and jejunum into the caecum, where it may be palpable on rectal examination as a firm tubular structure within the base of the caecum.

Ileo-ileal intussusceptions result in only partial obstruction of the lumen and minimal vascular impairment. They are characterized by sudden onset of moderately severe pain, which subsides within 8–12 hours, thereafter becoming mild and intermittent. This state of affairs may persist for several weeks, during which time considerable muscular hypertrophy of the wall of several metres of small intestine oral to the obstruction develops in response to the partial occlusion of the lumen at the site of intussusception.

Ileocaecal intussusceptions have a greater tendency to cause complete obstruction from their inception.

The average length of jejunal intussusceptions is 50–70 cm, but they can be considerably longer if the mesentery is torn. Owing to the pull of the involved mesentery, the intussusception takes on a screw-like concavity at its mesenteric border. As more and more mesentery is drawn in there is progressive interference with venous drainage, leading to congestion, oedema and haemorrhage and, finally, infarction and necrosis of the intussusceptum. Complete obstruction occurs very early on, and sudden onset of severe abdominal pain is always a feature of this type of obstruction.

Reduction of intussusceptions should be attempted before correction is initiated. Most ileo-ileal and some ileocaecal intussusceptions can be reduced. Although the short length of bowel wall involved in ileo-ileal intussusceptions does not undergo infarction, there is inevitably a degree of stricture present, which can be satisfactorily bypassed by side-to-side ileocaecal anastomosis proximal to the obstruction. Resection of intestine involved in ileocaecal intussusceptions is always necessary following reduction. Continuity is restored by side-to-side jejunocaecostomy. Where the intussusception is irreducible, the intestine is transected proximal to the point of invagination and a jejunocaecostomy performed. The distal ileal stump is inverted into the caecum. Alternatively, the invaginated bowel may be removed via a caecotomy (Freeman, 1997). Resection of intussuscepted jejunum is much easier following reduction. However, if this is not possible due to the length and friability of the invaginated bowel, it has to be resected *in situ*. Particular care must be taken in these cases to ensure that all the vessels in the affected mesentery are identified and ligated.

Pedunculated lipomas

Pedunculated lipomas are a common cause of strangulation obstruction in older horses; most animals affected are 12 years or more. Suspended on a mesenteric pedicle, they have the potential to wrap around a segment of small intestine which can vary in length from 25 cm to several metres, producing closed loop strangulation.

Pedunculated lipomas are a frequent cause of strangulating intestinal obstruction in older horses, but large lipomas attached at the mesenteric attachment to the gut can cause simple compression of the intestine, requiring no more than removal of the lipoma at surgery by sectioning its pedicle.

Clinical signs are similar to other forms of strangulating obstruction of the small intestine. The obstruction is characterized by acute unrelenting pain. Endotoxaemia and resulting cardiovascular deterioration is rapid, reflecting the severe vascular obstruction and rapidly developing necrosis of the intestine brought about by the tightly constricting pedicle.

The strangulated bowel is freed by cutting the avascular pedicle. This frequently has to be performed blindly deep within the abdominal cavity, using blunt-ended scissors. The devitalized gut is resected and an appropriate anastomosis performed. The bowel oral to the strangulation is frequently distended, and often will not function for several days after the resection is performed.

Small intestinal volvulus

Volvulus is produced by a 180° or more rotation of a segment of jejunum on its own mesentery. The length of intestine incorporated in a volvulus varies considerably. As more intestine (both proximal and distal) is drawn into the volvulus, twisting of the mesentery continues producing constriction of the intestine and its blood supply, resulting in strangulation obstruction with all its pathophysiological consequences. The distal limit of a volvulus is frequently the terminal ileum, because of its relatively fixed position at the ileocaecal junction. Lesions that predispose to volvulus include infarction, adhesions and fibrous bands, and congenital remnants of a mesodiverticular band or Meckel's diverticulum. Volvulus nodosus is a form of volvulus involving the distal jejunum and ileum and characterized by the formation of a 'knot', which progressively tightens by peristalsis and gas formation in the strangulated loop. It occurs most frequently in the foal. Usually, 30–150 cm of small intestine are affected.

Large intestine

The causes of large intestine ileus or obstruction are listed in Table 4.2. The signs of large intestinal obstruction include gas accumulation, in contrast to the fluid sequestration observed in the small intestine. The resulting clinical signs include tympany, abdominal distension and varying degrees of pain depending on the distension or vascular compromise.

Table 4.2 Large intestine obstruction

Simple obstruction	Impaction	Caecum
		Large colon
		Small colon/rectum
	Colonic displacement	Left dorsal
		Right dorsal
		Retroflexion
Strangulation obstruction	Volvulus	Caecum
		Large colon
	Intussusception	Caeco-caecal
		Caecocolic
		Small colon
Non-strangulating infarction		

Caecal impaction

There is no known cause for caecal dysfunction with distension. Caecal impaction is seen in two forms. In one form the caecum contains firm dry ingesta, which may fill the viscus or be more localized to the overhanging cranial part of the base of the caecum. In the second form, the caecum is immobile and markedly distended with ingesta of a relatively fluid consistency. Caecal impaction comprised 1.7 per cent of the cases in the Bolshoi study (White, 1990), and had a mortality rate of 43 per cent, mostly due to rupture. No specific cause is identified when the problem arises in horses on a normal hay and grain diet. Caecal impaction is a recognized problem in horses that are hospitalized, particularly those undergoing surgery unrelated to the alimentary tract. Musculoskeletal disease and therapy with non-steroidal anti-inflammatory drugs appear to be other contributory factors.

Horses with caecal impaction have mild to moderate intermittent pain. Intestinal sounds are reduced, and the heart rate varies with the degree of distension and stretching of the caecal wall. Rectally, the caecum (including the base) can be felt to be full of firm ingesta, which can just be indented with the finger. Dehydration occurs only slowly over several days. The protein in peritoneal fluid, which initially is normal, increases as the impaction becomes established. With caecal dysfunction the pain is often severe when associated with severe distension of the caecum, which can lead to mural ischaemia and rupture. Correspondingly, changes in cardiovascular parameters and peritoneal fluid are more marked. On rectal examination, the caecum feels similar to tympany but is pulled cranially by the weight of the food material and fluid.

Medical treatment should be employed for dehydrated impactions if possible, and is usually effective if the impaction is diagnosed early. All food should be withheld. Large volumes of intravenous fluid (2–4 l/hr) and 6–8 l of water orally every 2–3 hrs offer the best chance of success. Magnesium sulphate (1 g/kg once daily for 3 days) or dioctyl sodium sulfosuccinate (10–20 mg/kg) diluted in water and administered by stomach tube are preferable to administration of mineral oil, which is less effective than in large colon impactions because it can pass straight into the colon without penetrating the caecal mass. Pain may be controlled using flunixin meglumine, preferably at the lower dosage of 0.5 mg/kg. Because of the risk of caecal rupture, the horse must be monitored closely. If pain cannot be controlled or if changes in peritoneal fluid indicate bowel ischaemia, surgery should be carried out without delay.

Evacuation of impacted material can be carried out at laparotomy by lavage via an enterotomy near the apex of the caecum. However, in horses with severe impaction, recurrence of the problem is often complicated by rupture. Therefore, when compromise of normal caecal function or emptying is anticipated or has already been encountered, the caecum should be by-passed with an ileocolostomy. The ileum is transected and both ends closed with inverting sutures. The proximal end is then anastomosed side-to-side to the right ventral colon. This technique provides a better chance of permanent success than the alternatives of caecocolic anastomosis or ileocolostomy without transecting the ileum. None of these techniques is appropriate if the viability of the caecum has been compromised. In these cases, a partial or complete typhlectomy is the only alternative to euthanasia.

Chronic, recurrent caecal impaction over a period of several months is occasionally encountered, associated with muscular hypertrophy of the base of the caecum, which partially obstructs the caecocolic orifice. This hypertrophy can be demonstrated ultrasonographically. The obstruction can be relieved by enlarging the caecocolic orifice via a right flank approach and removal of the eighteenth rib (Huskamp, 1998b); alternatively, the caecum may be bypassed by means of an ileocolostomy.

Large colon impaction

Food impaction

Impaction of food in the large colon constitutes the most common form of colonic obstruction, and is therefore a frequent cause of colic. It is not well established what causes the impaction. Factors thought to contribute include coarseness of feed, poor dentition, inadequate mastication, decreased water intake, or major dysfunction that disrupts bowel motility. Impaction occurs at two sites of narrowing; the pelvic flexure and the transverse colon. At these sites, where motor centres can induce retention to aid mixing of food, natural retention of ingesta appears to predominate, over-riding the normal aboral flow. Changing the horse's activity level from routine exercise to stall confinement, such as occurs with injury, appears to increase the risk of impaction.

Clinical signs and diagnosis
Horses with feed impactions usually present with mild to moderate intermittent colic and decreased faecal output. Faeces are often hard, dry and mucus covered. Decreased food intake progresses to complete refusal to eat. If water intake is also decreased, signs of dehydration will develop. Initially intestinal sounds are variable and may, with time,

continue to decrease until absent. Auscultation at a time when the horse is exhibiting pain frequently reveals peristaltic movement, indicating increased pressure against the obstruction. The amount of pain will increase with complete obstruction or pressure necrosis of bowel around the impaction. Pulse rate, mucous membrane colour and respiratory rate are generally normal until dehydration and bowel degeneration occur. Gastric reflux is absent in all but exceptional cases. Peritoneal fluid is initially normal, but severe distension leads to an increase in protein. An increase in white blood cells indicates bowel necrosis. Rectal examination frequently reveals a firm mass of ingesta in the pelvic flexure or ventral colon. The pelvic flexure may lie within the pelvic canal, extending caudally as far as the peritoneal reflection. Making a note of the extent and firmness of the impaction will help evaluate progress following treatment. Complete obstruction of the colon causes gas to accumulate gradually in the intestines, causing caecal and colon distension, and in transverse colon impactions this will be the only abnormality palpable.

Treatment

If diagnosed early and treated effectively, most feed impactions respond to conservative medical therapy comprising oral laxatives, mild analgesics and intravenous or oral fluids. If allowed access to food, the horses will continue to eat and thereby add to the amount of impacted ingesta. Therefore, food should be completely restricted until the impaction is relieved, but water should be provided *ad lib*. If bedded on straw, the horse should be removed to a stall with peat, shavings or paper bedding, or muzzled. Laxatives such as mineral oil are vital for relieving impactions, and 3–5 l of mineral oil may be administered by nasogastric tube to a 450 kg horse over 12–24 hours.

Controlling the relatively mild discomfort is not difficult, but the need to retain and encourage the gut motility necessary to facilitate softening and propulsion of the impacted material requires that the choice of analgesic and dose rate be considered carefully. Flunixin meglumine, which does not alter intestinal motility, used in as low a dose as possible (0.1–0.2 mg/kg) is usually adequate.

Passage of large amounts of soft, oily faeces is indicative that the impaction is clearing. How soon after treatment this will commence and how long it will take to clear completely depends on the firmness of the ingesta, the length of colon impacted and the length of time the condition had been present prior to treatment. The average time taken to clear the impaction in a study by White and Dabareiner (1997) was 48 hours.

Resistant cases will require further administration of mineral oil, but benefit most from 'over-hydration' using a balanced electrolyte solution intravenously at a rate of 40–60 l per 24-hour period, which helps to soften the mass and maintain motility. This will usually abort the need for surgery, but may take 3–5 days to clear the impaction. During this period the horse should be examined regularly, including a rectal examination, to monitor progress and check on its cardiovascular status. Continued pain, increasing heart rate and changes in peritoneal fluid are indications for surgery, which should not be delayed, to avoid further compromise of the bowel wall.

Sand impaction

Horses on pasture in areas of sandy soil are at risk of accumulating sand in the colon and, eventually, suffering episodes of colic. Horses that have short or non-existent grass on their pasture or inadequate roughage in their diet are prone to consume sand while attempting to gather bits of feed from the ground. Some, especially foals, may deliberately eat sand. Locations with a high incidence include Florida, California and Michigan. In the UK the condition is uncommon, but it is encountered during periods of prolonged dry weather in horses grazing in coastal or river estuary pastures.

Clinical signs

Horses with sand impaction tend to present with the same signs as horses with ingesta impactions. The intermittent pain caused by the weight of sand often prompts the horse to lie on its back or stretch out for long periods, in an attempt to reduce the tension on the intestine. Because of the abrasive nature of sand, mucosal irritation and damage may lead to diarrhoea. This inflammatory response, associated with accumulation of sufficient volume of sand, can result in colonic rupture. Rectal examination often allows palpation of firm sand in the colon. However, sand that has accumulated in the distal right colon or transverse colon can be difficult to detect. Coarse sand may be felt as 'grit' with the fingers during palpation, but fine sand is frequently not palpable. Confirmation of excessive amounts of sand can be achieved by inverting a rectal glove over four to six balls of faeces and filling it with water. After mixing the faeces into a slurry the sleeve is suspended for several minutes, allowing the sand to settle into the fingers of the glove.

When the ventral abdomen is auscultated, the movement of sand within the intestine may be heard as pouring sand (Ragle *et al.*, 1989). Peritoneal fluid is often normal, or may show a slight rise in protein. Due to the weight of the colon, accidental penetration with the needle or cannula can easily occur. Abdominal radiography can reveal sand impactions in foals, ponies and miniature horses. Similarly, ultrasonography can provide images consistent with accumulation of coarse sandy material in the large colon.

Treatment

The same laxatives used for treating feed impactions may also be used for conservative therapy of sand impaction. The laxative of choice for sand impactions is Psyllium hydrophile muciloid flakes, at a dosage of 500 g per 450 kg in 9 l (2 gallons) of water, administered by nasogastric tube. The gel formed lubricates and binds with the sand, moving it distally and helping to clear the impaction. This treatment is normally repeated at least twice, at 2–3 day intervals. The faeces should be monitored closely for the clearance of sand. Although the signs of colic may cease, the complete removal of the sand is never confirmed.

Magnesium sulphate may also be used to clear the sand, at a dose of 1 mg/kg in 3–4 l of water, via a stomach tube. This dose can be repeated for 3 consecutive days, and then again after 5–7 days for resistant cases.

As with other forms of impaction, surgery is indicated if there is unrelenting pain, a palpable mass of sand in the colon, changes in the peritoneal fluid indicating degeneration of bowel, or deterioration in the horse's condition. The sand must be removed by thorough lavage of the colon via an enterotomy near the pelvic flexure.

Where horses are kept in an environment that predisposes them to ingestion of sand, preventative measures should be taken – including feeding off the ground, grazing on pastures with adequate growth, or feeding of hay when the pastures are short. Preventing sand colic has been attempted with daily or weekly feeding of Psyllium or methyl-cellulose. Fifty grams (one cup) twice daily has been prescribed, though the efficacy has been questioned. Though this may be effective, the best way to prevent sand colic is to prevent sand intake by appropriate feeding of pasture and roughage without sand contamination.

Large colon (ascending colon) displacements

The horse is anatomically predisposed to a variety of colonic malpositions. The large colon of the horse is voluminous compared to other species, and comprises a long loop that is folded at the sternal, pelvic and diaphragmatic flexures to fit within the confines of the abdomen. The origin of the right ventral colon and terminal part of the right dorsal colon are fixed in position by attachments to the caecum, transverse colon and adjacent structures, but most of the colon is potentially mobile, restricted only by its size and contents.

The entire ascending colon is supplied by branches of the cranial mesenteric artery, which enter the colon through the attachment of the caecum to the dorsal wall. The vessels enter at the site where torsions commonly originate, thus predisposing the colon to vascular compromise because of blood vessel compression.

Left dorsal displacement (LDDC, nephrosplenic entrapment)

Displacement of the ascending colon between the dorsal abdominal wall, the left kidney, the nephrosplenic ligament and the dorsal border of the spleen is seen predominantly in mature horses, especially large geldings; mares, small horses and foals are seldom affected.

The entrapment may be complete or partial, depending upon whether the edge of the spleen is laterodorsal (complete) or ventral (partial) to the displaced bowel. The spleen is usually enlarged. The loop of colon draped over the tightly stretched nephrosplenic ligament is almost always rotated through 180° along its long axis so that the ventral colon lies above the dorsal colon on the ligaments. The large colon may herniate into the nephrosplenic space as far as the middle of the right dorsal and ventral colon. The diaphragmatic and sternal flexures are frequently displaced between the stomach and the left lobe of the liver.

Left dorsal displacement generally takes a protracted course, compared to conditions causing vascular compromise. However, in rare cases it takes a peracute course, leading to shock within 3–6 hours, and can be confused with large colon volvulus.

The majority of cases show mild to moderate pain. There is little or no rise in pulse rate, and signs of shock are generally absent. A poor response to analgesic and spasmolytic drugs indicates continued obstruction. Auscultation of the abdomen reveals tympanitic sounds, but only rarely are borborygmi absent. Positive gastric reflux is frequently present, and it is important routinely to pass a nasogastric tube before anaesthetizing the horse. Abdominal paracentesis reveals clear fluid, but frank haemorrhage may indicate puncture of the apex of the spleen. Rectal examination is the most useful diagnostic aid.

The treatment options include surgical correction, rolling, and con-servative medical management. During surgical correction, repositioning is carried out via a 20–30 cm ventral midline incision. Confirmation of the entrapment is usually possible at this stage, but gross distension and oedema of the colon may make it difficult. Spontaneous correction may have taken place during anaesthesia and transfer to the operating table.

The pelvic flexure is located and carefully lifted through the abdominal incision. A significantly shorter length than normal of left colon can be mobilized. There is often oedema of the mesocolon and slight mural oedema. Needle suction is used to decompress the colon of gas and in some cases, where a greater degree of vascular occlusion is present, it may be necessary to evacuate its contents through an enterotomy incision near the pelvic flexure before attempting repositioning.

The colon is restored to its correct position by simultaneous rotation of the spleen medially and ventrally, and elevation of the colon in a dorsolateral and cranial direction. To carry out this manoeuvre, the surgeon is best positioned on the right side of the horse.

Repositioning can be achieved quickly and simply, except in those cases in which the colon contains a large amount of food material. Here, the size of the colon makes it necessary to elevate it by degrees rather than in a single movement. Once freed, it is drawn from its position between the stomach and the liver. The entire length of colon can now be mobilized. The site of compression at the nephrosplenic ligament is usually identified by slight indentation and some serosal petechiation. These changes, together with oedema of the mesocolon, confirm that entrapment had been present in cases in which the colon is found free during surgical exploration. The colon is returned to the abdomen and placed in its normal position. The spleen, which rapidly reduces in size once the entrapment is corrected, is checked to ensure that it is in its correct position against the abdominal wall.

Several methods of rolling have been described (Boening and von

Saldern, 1986; Kalsbeek, 1989), but the principle is the same in each. A short-acting intravenous anaesthetic such as xylazine/ketamine can be used. The use of phenylnephrine (1–3 µg/kg per minute for 15 minutes) by intravenous infusion just prior to anaesthesia to contract the spleen has been described as an adjunct to the rolling technique (Hardy *et al.*, 1994). More recently, its use in the conscious horse has been described. The horse's heart rate, packed cell volume and blood pressure are checked during infusion of phenylephrine 3–6 µg/kg over a 15 minute period, following which the horse is exercised on a long lunge line for 30–45 minutes (Johnston, 1996). When rolling is employed, the horse is first positioned in right lateral recumbency. In this position the spleen is uppermost and should fall away from the body wall, releasing the constriction on the left colon. The horse is then rolled into dorsal recumbency, with or without elevation of the hindquarters, and the abdomen is rocked from side to side. After 1–2 minutes, the horse is rolled through left lateral recumbency, to sternal recumbency, and back into right lateral recumbency. This procedure may be repeated several times if necessary.

The nephrosplenic space may be checked by rectal palpation for absence of the large colon before the horse is allowed to recover from anaesthesia.

The principle candidates for rolling are horses with mild to moderate pain without severe distension. Failure to correct a left dorsal displacement by rolling is not in itself an indication for surgery. Because surgery may be necessary, however, rolling should not be performed unless a surgical facility is readily available. Complications of rolling include failure due to misdiagnosis, inability to correct the entrapment and creation of other displacements (Sivula, 1990), including large colon volvulus. Surgery is indicated in all cases of colon displacement with evidence of vascular impairment.

The rolling technique is not recommended in the pregnant mare.

The most important features of medical treatment are to maintain hydration with intravenous fluids, withhold feed and monitor closely for evidence of pain and systemic deterioration. If pain is mild and transient, analgesics may be used.

Conservative therapy of this type takes 48–72 hours to be successful. Pain will recur if the horse is fed before the displacement corrects itself. If the horse becomes painful or systemic parameters deteriorate, other measures must be taken.

Accurate assessment of non-surgical management of left dorsal displacement is difficult because a diagnosis based on rectal examination is not 100 per cent accurate, even when supported by ultrasonography. Therefore, some forms of colon tympany or some undetermined displacements may be treated in this manner with success. Conversely, some horses only diagnosed as left dorsal displacement at surgery may have been candidates for non-surgical management. When signs persist, surgery is the best option so that serious disease is diagnosed and corrected early.

Prognosis

If the condition is recognized during the first 72 hours in mild cases, or 12 hours in peracute cases, the prognosis is very good. The very few cases that do not survive usually have infarction of the colon, which leads to rupture during correction. Occasionally recurrence of the problem may occur, but the incidence is low.

Right dorsal displacement of the colon (RDDC)

This form of colonic displacement is much less common than left dorsal displacement. The large colon passes between the right body wall and the caecum, initially in a cranial to caudal direction. It then displaces further cranially, until the pelvic flexure reaches the diaphragm. There is concomitant bending or flexion of the colon originating at the transverse colon. In addition, right dorsal displacement may be accompanied by a colon volvulus. The location of the torsion is rarely the same as that of the flexion. At the site of flexion, the dorsal and ventral parts of the colon are partially occluded. If torsion is present there is further occlusion, which will be complete in cases of 360° volvulus and will be accompanied by strangulation changes.

Right dorsal displacement is seen in large-framed horses that are usually housed at the time the problem is seen. Although the course of the disease may be fairly protracted, with mild attacks of colic alternating with apparent complete recovery, in most cases it is acute and violent.

In the relatively mild, protracted cases, there is some distension of the right flank due to colonic tympany. The blood values are initially normal and there is negative gastric reflux.

In the more acute cases, signs of shock are evident. Abdominal distension is considerably greater, the packed cell volume is increased and considerable volumes of fluid may be obtained on passage of a nasogastric tube. Rectal examination often reveals the colon coursing to the right of the caecum.

There is no documented successful treatment of RDDC by rolling, and surgical correction carried out via a ventral midline incision is the only option. The pelvic flexure is located near the diaphragm and exteriorized, and an enterotomy performed to allow the colon to be emptied of gas and ingesta. After closure of the enterotomy incision, the right ventral colon is identified by tracing the lateral band of the caecum to the caecocolic fold, and traction carefully applied to bring the remainder of the colon from around the caecum so that it can be returned to its correct position.

Provided the condition is recognized early in its course and surgery is performed promptly, the prognosis is very good. Prognosis is not so good for those cases where colon volvulus has affected the bowel's viability.

Cranial displacement of the pelvic flexure

Cranial displacements of the pelvic flexure lead to kinking or flexion of the dorsal and ventral colon, with narrowing of the intestinal lumen causing a partial obstruction. It usually develops secondary to tympany and impaction.

The initial clinical signs are mild. Rectal examination reveals tympany of the colon, but the pelvic flexure cannot be palpated. Conservative treatment is not always successful, and surgical correction becomes necessary when the obstruction is not relieved during medical treatment.

Large colon volvulus

The incidence of volvulus (also called torsion) of the large colon has been reported to range from 11–17 per cent of horses treated surgically for colic, and accounts for nearly 40 per cent of obstructions involving the large colon. There appears to be no breed predisposition. Adult horses and older brood mares just before or after parturition have the highest incidence. In Kentucky, horses with colon volvulus comprise 26–34 per cent of the surgical colic cases, of which 87 per cent are mares (Embertson, 1997).

Regardless of the predisposing causes for large colon volvulus, mares that have had one episode stand approximately a 15 per cent chance of a second occurrence (Fischer and Meagher, 1986). This is increased to approximately 80 per cent if the mare has had two or more episodes.

Volvulus that has progressed to a strangulation obstruction is the most devastating form of colic in horses. The overall survival rates reported are low (21–42 per cent), despite improvements in surgical techniques and post-operative care. This is due largely to delay in carrying out surgery, resulting in advanced ischaemic damage to the colon and severe endotoxic and hypovolaemic shock. If surgery is carried out within 2 hours of the onset of colic, correction of the volvulus can be performed relatively easily, with a much higher survival rate.

Rotation occurs about the long axis of the double loop of dorsal and ventral colon, usually in a clockwise direction with respect to the root of the mesentery when viewed from behind. In doing so, the right dorsal colon moves laterally while rotating ventrally and the right ventral colon moves medially while rotating dorsally. A volvulus of 90–180° may reduce spontaneously, or progress to 270–720°. A volvulus of greater than 270° results in vascular obstruction, which can rapidly lead to severe colonic devitalization. The volvulus may involve only the left dorsal and left ventral colons where they merge with the diaphragmatic and sternal flexures. The majority of these are non-strangulating, and are sometimes described as being partial. However, most volvuluses are strangulating and occur at the base of the colon just cranial to the caecum, although in some cases the caecum is also involved.

The exact cause of colonic volvulus is unknown. It is speculated that hypomotility due to pain, intestinal fatty acid content or electrolyte abnormalities may lead to bowel stasis and distension. Undesirable fermentation processes may lead to excessive gas formation and 'floating' of the larger ventral colon over the smaller dorsal colon along the entire length of the colon. Alternatively, the rotation could commence at the pelvic flexure and be transmitted like a coil in a rope until it reaches the base.

At the site of constriction, the loops of colon are entwined in spiral fashion. The degree of circulatory impairment depends not only on the degree of torsion but also on the distension of the colon with food material and gas, which exacerbates obstruction of the blood vessels by the longitudinal bands. Occlusion of the veins with a sustained arterial supply leads to severe congestive hyperaemia and extravasation, producing severe oedema of the bowel wall and mesocolon. If both arterial and venous obstruction is present from the outset, the serosa appears grey and there is minimal oedema. Mucosal necrosis develops quickly, leading to profound endotoxaemia. Gross tympany causes respiratory difficulty and further circulatory embarrassment by exerting pressure on the great vessels.

The clinical signs depend on the degree of volvulus, the duration of vascular occlusion and length of colon involved. Most cases present with sudden onset of severe and unrelenting pain, and their behaviour may be so violent and unpredictable that a thorough examination may be impossible. Systemic deterioration is rapid, with a rapid weak pulse, poor peripheral perfusion and a high PCV, which may rise to above 60 in just 2–3 hours. There is marked abdominal distension, and the grossly enlarged colon is palpable on rectal examination. The wall is thick and oedematous and the colon is usually forced back into the pelvic inlet, although in rare cases of volvulus unaccompanied by significant gas accumulation it may be displaced so far anteriorly that, in large horses, it can no longer be reached *per rectum*.

The characteristic violent behaviour, tympany, peracute course and rectal findings enable a prompt diagnosis of colonic torsion to be made, and it is often apparent that immediate surgery is indicated within an hour or two of onset. In exceptional cases the course is more protracted, and can extend over several days. In these cases, the partial obstruction allows the passage of gas through the twisted portion of bowel, thereby preventing tympany. The gut wall and mesocolon are oedematous, but necrosis of the mucosa is absent initially. Affected horses are anorexic and suffer mild bouts of colic. The rectal findings of oedematous colon establish the diagnosis.

Surgical correction of colonic torsion must be carried out as early as possible. Anaesthetic management of these patients can be a major challenge. Abdominal distension and the compromised metabolic state of these horses predispose them to ventilation–perfusion mismatches, resulting in hypercapnia and inadequate oxygenation. Severe colonic distension results in a hypotensive crisis due to inadequate ventilation and impaired venous return. Further haemodynamic compromise may occur when endotoxin and other mediators are released upon correcting the torsion.

A long ventral midline incision may be required to allow easier manipulation of the distended colon, which requires great care to avoid splitting of the oedematous and often friable colon wall. Gaseous decompression can be easily achieved by needle puncture and suction before the left colon is brought through the abdominal incision. A pelvic flexure enterotomy and evacuation of the colon contents may be necessary to facilitate correction of the volvulus. There is less risk of rupture of the colon if the counter-rotation is performed with the colon within the abdominal cavity. Accurate assessment of colon viability is important but difficult, because there is no reliable, easily applicable intra-operative method available. Visual evaluation of the serosal surface is the most convenient but least accurate method, because the colour may return to almost normal after correction of the volvulus. Histo-pathological examination of frozen sections and assessment of the extent of mucosal necrosis (Snyder *et al.*, 1990) is probably the most accurate, but is time-consuming and has very limited availability. Consequently, viability is usually determined on the basis of mesenteric, serosal and mucosal colour, with special emphasis on whether there is mural haemorrhage at the site of the enterotomy used to evacuate the colon contents. Necrotic mucosa and lack of haemorrhage at this site, together with a haematocrit value in excess of 50 per cent and body temperature greater than 38.9°C (102°F), indicate a poor chance of survival.

Caecal intussusception

Caecal intussusceptions take one of two forms. Following the initial invagination of the apex of the caecum, the intussusception may be limited to the caecum (caeco-caecal), or may continue until most of the caecum has passed through the caecocolic orifice into the right ventral colon (caecocolic). While their cause is generally unknown, a significant number of cases have heavy tapeworm infestations. Clinical signs of the condition are dependent on which type is present.

Caeco-caecal intussusceptions do not completely obstruct the flow of ingesta, and clinical signs therefore commence as a moderately severe colic and subside to a mild continuous type. The horse appears depressed and has decreased gut motility. Physiologically, the patient deteriorates rather slowly.

Caecocolic intussusception, on the other hand, is much more likely to obstruct the passage of ingesta. Affected animals show a moderate colic, which becomes more severe as the small intestine distends. They have very little motility, and eventually show gastric reflux. Physiologically, they deteriorate more rapidly. Both conditions will result in serosanguinous peritoneal fluid. On rectal examination, failure to identify the caecum and the presence of a firm, painful mass in the right dorsal quadrant suggests the presence of a caecal intussusception. If not corrected surgically, even non-obstructing intussusceptions result in intermittent mild colic and progressive weight loss over a period of weeks or months.

At laparotomy the 'absence' of caecum is confirmed, but careful palpation within the abdominal cavity will identify the point of invagination. Caeco-caecal invaginations, and those that have only very recently progressed to caecocolic intussusception, can be reduced and the strangulated portion of the caecum resected. However, when almost total invagination has taken place, gross oedema of the caecum makes reduction through the small caecocolic orifice impossible. In these cases, the right ventral colon may be incised and the bulk of the invaginated caecum amputated. Alternatively, the intussusception may be left *in situ* and an ileocolostomy performed. However, unlike reducible caecal intussusceptions, irreducible invaginations carry a poor prognosis.

Small colon

Retained meconium

Meconium is a mucilaginous material found in the intestine of the foetus at full term, comprising glandular secretions of the gastrointestinal tract, amniotic fluid swallowed by the foetus and cellular debris. It is greenish black to light brown in colour, and has little odour. Ordinarily, meconium is moved along the gastrointestinal tract into the colon and rectum before birth. Ingestion of colostrum may promote gastrointestinal activity and aid passage. Meconium usually begins to be evacuated from the neonatal foal within 3 hours of birth. Many foals strain to pass meconium, and nearly all pass meconium by 48 hours of age.

Meconium retention refers to the difficulty in passage of meconium rather than the time over which it is passed. Male foals appear to be more commonly affected, and this has been considered to be due to the narrower pelvic canal. In the Bolshoi study (White, 1990), meconium retention was the most common cause of rectal obstruction and accounted for 0.8 per cent of cases. In the same study, the mortality for this condition was 15.2 per cent.

Clinical signs

The clinical signs of meconium retention include restlessness, attempts to defecate, straining to defecate, tail swishing, tail elevation and disinterest in sucking. Advanced signs are colic, lying down and getting up, rolling and lying upside down, which are associated with distension of bowel proximal to the obstruction.

Diagnosis

Diagnosis is based on clinical signs and palpation of a firm mass at the entrance to the pelvis with a well-lubricated finger inserted into the rectum, associated with absence of yellow milk stool. A positive response to the administration of enemas is further confirmation of the problem. In severe cases that are slow to respond, abdominal palpation may reveal firm faecal material masses in the small colon. Abdominal radiography will confirm the extent of the obstruction and demonstrate the accumulation of gas and fluid oral to it.

Treatment

The preferred method of treatment is the administration of enemas, and most simple impactions of the rectum and distal small colon can be cleared by this means. Manual extraction should be avoided due to the risk of tearing or perforating the rectum. The routine administration of enemas on farms by grooms is accompanied by some degree of risk. Rough or frequent tubing can cause rectal irritation and oedema, prompting tenesmus, which can confuse the picture.

Enemas should preferably be administered by gravity flow, but can be given safely by the gentle use of a Higginson's enema syringe. A variety of enemas have been used with variable success, and 100–500 ml of a mild soapy water enema, which lubricates, reduces surface tension and softens the mass, is as effective as any. Commercial phosphate enemas have been used with success but, due to the risk of hyperphosphataemia, should not be used more than two or three times. Dioctyl sodium sulfosuccinate (DSS) (10 ml of 5 per cent solution diluted in warm water) and acetyl cysteine (8 g added to 200 ml of water containing 20 g sodium bicarbonate) are other useful alternatives, but repeated use of DSS can cause mucosal irritation.

Low doses of analgesics may be required to control pain. Concretions that do not respond to conservative treatment seem to be more common in foals with underlying problems, e.g. prematurity or respiratory distress. Decreased gut motility and/or dehydration may be contributory factors.

Additional therapy will be required in the form of 200–500 ml of mineral oil or DSS 10–15 ml (5 per cent) diluted in 200 ml of water by nasogastric tube, and intravenous fluids to overcome the dehydration.

Fortunately, colonic concretions only rarely require surgical correction. After surgical exposure of the impaction, digital massage to break down the mass and gentle flushing of the rectum and affected portion of the colon are preferable to enterotomy because this is less likely to lead to post-operative adhesions.

Impaction

Impaction of the small colon is rare, but is still one of the most common diseases affecting the small colon (Edwards, 1997). Ponies appear to be at greater risk compared to other breeds. Salmonella spp. can be cultured from 10–25 per cent of horses with this disease. The cause of impaction of considerable lengths of small colon with dehydrated ingesta is not known, but stasis similar to that of the large colon is suspected. Other suggested contributory factors include decreased water supply, poor quality roughage and inadequate mastication.

Focal obstruction of the small colon by enteroliths, faecoliths, phytobezoars and foreign bodies such as nylon materials and rubber fencing can cause secondary impaction.

The signs of small colon impaction are mild to moderate pain, abdominal distension, a tubular mass of firm ingesta in the small colon on rectal examination and, in a minority of cases, nasogastric reflux (Ruggles and Ross, 1991). The peritoneal fluid may have an increase in protein concentration, depending on the duration of the impaction.

Treatment may be medical or surgical. A higher long-term recovery rate has been reported in horses treated medically by administration of mineral oil and saline by nasogastric tube and vigorous intravenous therapy to 'over-hydrate' the horse in an effort to hydrate the impacting mass (Ruggles and Ross, 1991). Flunixin meglumine at 0.5 mg/kg is administered two to four times daily. Saline enemas administered by a lubricated nasogastric tube in the standing horse should only be considered when the impaction is present at the rectum. The volume of saline infused must be measured and administered very slowly to prevent rectal tearing. Surgical treatment should be carried out without delay if pain cannot be controlled, if there is increasing abdominal distension and if the protein concentration and WBC count in the peritoneal fluid indicate vascular compromise of the bowel wall. At laparotomy, most of the small colon is found to be impacted uniformly with digesta, creating a tubular structure with none of the usual sacculations. Frequently, the impaction terminates at the pelvic inlet. The impacted mass may be injected with fluid (Meagher, 1974), or may be cleared by retrograde flushing through a tube introduced via the anus. This procedure must be carried out with the utmost care to minimize hyperaemia and oedema of the small colon, which predisposes to a recurrence of impaction. When most of the small colon is involved the author prefers to flush in both directions through an enterotomy located midway along the impacted segment, thus reducing the amount of handling to which the distal part is subjected. Feeding a low-fibre, high-energy diet such as a complete pelleted feed after surgery is recommended (White and Dabareiner, 1997).

Enteroliths can cause obstruction of the large, transverse and small colons. The incidence is higher in particular regions, such as California and Florida in the US. They can occur whenever a nidus for precipitation is present and the appropriate proportion of magnesium is present in the diet.

Clinical signs

Signs are similar to those of colon obstruction. Pain may be severe if the stone becomes lodged in the transverse colon or small colon and if the obstruction becomes complete, preventing gas from escaping from the colons. The heart rate is mildly elevated, unless there is severe distension. Gastric reflux may also be seen, apparently due to stasis of the entire gastrointestinal tract.

Diagnosis

The enterolith may be felt *per rectum* if it has passed far enough aborally in the small colon, or it may be possible to ballot it in the transverse colon just in front of the mesenteric stalk. In some cases horses will have repeated bouts of colic, apparently from intermittent obstruction. Radiographs of the abdomen can be used to diagnose enterolithiasis. The technique requires a 600 mA machine, rare earth screens and 160 kVp (Rose and Rose, 1987). Four quadrants of the abdomen are examined. In areas of high risk, this procedure may be used to identify enteroliths before they cause obstruction.

Treatment

Though some enteroliths will pass through the small colon, most stones that cause obstruction must be removed surgically. Surgery involves locating the stone through a ventral midline incision and completing an enterotomy at the site of obstruction. If the stone is located in the transverse colon, it is moved back into the large colon. This may be facilitated by flushing fluid via a tube inserted through the rectum and small colon, or by injecting saline adjacent to the transverse colon to dilate the intestine to help free the enterolith.

A high rate of survival is reported with surgical removal of enteroliths. Though there can be bruising of the intestinal wall, there is rarely infarction of the bowel unless the stone has caused pressure necrosis over a long period of time.

Strangulation obstruction

Strangulation obstructions of the small colon are rare. Although the small colon has a relatively long mesentery, both incarceration and volvulus are rare. Rupture of the mesocolon with subsequent segmental ischaemic necrosis of the small colon has been recognized as a rare complication of parturition in the mare, either associated with rectal prolapse or as a result of direct trauma, possibly due to vigorous kicking movements that occur during extension of the foetal limbs as rotation into the dorsal position for delivery takes place. Strangulation by a pedunculated lipoma in old horses does occur, but is much less common than obstruction of the small intestine. Intussusception has been recorded, and segments of small colon can herniate through a variety of tissue layers. In foals, the colon can become strangulated in an umbilical hernia and, in mature and immature males, through an inguinal ring. Sites for strangulating hernias also include omental tears, tears in the uterine broad ligament, holes in the mesentery of the large colon and uterine and vaginal tears. Mural or submucosal haematomas occur in the small colon, producing a form of strangulation.

Peritonitis

Peritonitis is an inflammation of the mesothelial membrane that lines the peritoneal cavity and covers the intra-abdominal viscera, and is characterized by hyperaemia, peritoneal effusion and fibrin deposition, chemotactic phagocytosis and increased peritoneal permeability to toxins. It is usually, but not invariably, attended by signs of abdominal pain. Although it can be a primary disease entity, it is more commonly seen as a secondary complication associated with infectious (bacterial, viral, fungal or parasitic) or non-infectious (traumatic, chemical or neoplastic) stimuli (Table 4.3). In primary peritonitis the route of bacterial spread is not evident, but impaired defences may be involved. In secondary peritonitis, bacteria most commonly gain access to the peritoneal cavity following disruption of the integrity of the gastrointestinal tract or, less frequently, the urinogenital tract or abdominal wall. Prognostically it is important to know whether the infection is localized, spreading or diffuse, and whether the course of the problem is acute or chronic. Its severity is related to a number of factors, including the underlying problem, the nature of the infectious agent, the resistance of the host, the speed of recognition and intervention and the response to initial therapy. The inflammatory responses in peritonitis mobilize leucocytes and immunoglobulins and cause a profound relocation of proteins, fluid and electrolytes from plasma, which can lead to cardiovascular collapse. Fibrinolytic activity is depressed and fibrin is rapidly precipitated, either focally at the site of an intestinal perforation

Table 4.3 Causes of peritonitis

Infectious or septic	Non-septic	Parasitic	Traumatic	Iatrogenic
Surgical complications	Ruptured bladder, kidney or ureter	Parasitic larval migration	Penetrating abdominal wound	Rectal tear
• anastomosis failure	Chemical agents	Perforating lesions (ascarids, tapeworms)	Blunt abdominal trauma	Uterine perforation
• non-viable tissue	• bile			
• poor asepsis	• gastric juice		Breeding or foaling accident	• infusion
• excessive haemorrhage	• pancreatic juice	Verminous arteritis		• biopsy
• uncorrected or supervening obstructions			Ruptured diaphragm	• artificial insemination
• peritoneal irritants and foreign bodies	Foreign body			
	Neoplasia			Enterocentesis
	• abdominal			
Intestinal accidents with perforation	• ovarian			Caecal rochartization
Abdominal abscesses	Urolithiasis			
	Hepatitis			Liver biopsy
Uterine rupture or perforation	Gastric rupture			Laparoscopy procedure
Metritis				
Urachal infection				
Post-castration infection				
Enteritis				
Septicaemia				
Cholangitis				

or diffusely as in septic peritonitis or following major gastrointestinal leakage. Although initially of benefit by confining contamination and infection, these processes may become deleterious, resulting in hypovolaemia, hypoproteinaemia, reflex ileus with bowel distension, ischaemia of the bowel wall allowing absorption of bacteria and toxins, and adhesion formation. Death is due to a combination of factors, but shock is a common denominator. The events mentioned above, together with a progressive deterioration of body defence mechanisms, are translated into a progression of failures – cardiovascular, respiratory, adrenocortical and hepato-renal.

Clinical signs

The clinical features of peritonitis are extremely variable, depending on the aetiology, extent and duration of the disease.

Horses with peracute peritonitis (e.g. following gastric rupture) may be found dead or present with profound toxaemia, which rapidly leads to circulatory failure and death within 4–12 hours.

Those with acute diffuse peritonitis exhibit tachycardia, tachypnoea, congested to cyanotic mucous membranes, cold extremities, thready pulse, dehydration and depression. Although both visceral and parietal pain may be present, parietal pain, characterized by immobility, splinting of the abdominal wall and sensitivity to pressure, is usually the major contributor.

Horses with localized, subacute or chronic peritonitis show dullness, decreased appetite and progressive weight loss. Abdominal pain may be low-grade, intermittent or absent. Other signs include intermittent fever, variable bowel sounds and, in some cases, chronic diarrhoea.

Diagnosis

A definitive diagnosis of peritonitis can usually be made simply by examination of a peritoneal fluid sample for cytology and fluid protein. However, peritoneal fluid analysis does not permit diagnosis of the underlying cause of peritonitis, which may be very important in determining the treatment and prognosis.

The peritoneal fluid may be turbid and off-white in colour (suggesting a high white blood cell (WBC) count), homogeneously blood-stained (suggesting haemoperitoneum or intestinal infarction), or turbid and brown/green in colour (suggesting contamination with intestinal contents). The white cell count in acute peritonitis ($> 100\,000$ per mm^3) is higher than in chronic peritonitis ($20\,000$–$60\,000$ per mm^3). Early in the inflammatory process the elevated WBC count is due primarily to an increase in polymorphs, while in chronic cases there is an increase in mononuclear cells and macrophages. Peritoneal fluid protein concentration is significantly higher than normal. In addition to cytologic and biochemical analysis, samples should be submitted for Gram staining and bacterial culture with sensitivity testing. More than 60 per cent of septic peritonitis cases are due to mixed bacterial infections. Peritonitis is more difficult to diagnose after abdominal surgery, because manipulation of the bowel causes an elevation in peritoneal WBC and total protein content.

Further evaluation of the degree of severity of peritonitis depends on laboratory estimation of fluid and electrolyte balance, blood gas analysis and haematology. In peracute and acute peritonitis, there is leucopenia with neutropenia and a degenerative left shift. Protein sequestration and fluid exudation into the peritoneal cavity leads to hypoproteinaemia and dehydration. In acute peritonitis of longer duration and in localized or chronic peritonitis, the changes in total WBC count are less dramatic. A decrease in albumin/globulin ratio is frequently present.

The rectal findings in cases of peritonitis are variable. Contamination of the abdominal cavity with gastrointestinal contents results in a gritty feeling to the surface of the bowel. Free gas and increased peritoneal fluid tend to separate loops of distended bowel, giving an impression of more room and making examination easier. In mares with uterine rupture, a fibrinous adhesion may be noted over the affected area. Distended bowel or secondary impactions may be evident, while oedema of the wall of the large colon or caecum may indicate focal or more generalized infarction. In other cases, no abnormalities may be palpable. Ultrasonography and laparoscopy can be of diagnostic value. In foals, lateral standing radiographs may show fluid, ileus or free gas, which allows the cranial pole of the right kidney to be visualized.

Early exploratory laparotomy may be indicated for diagnostic, therapeutic and prognostic reasons, and is best performed while the horse is in reasonable condition. Where there is a spreading peritonitis from an uncontrolled source of contamination (e.g. perforated or infarcted bowel), operative surgery is mandatory if any life-saving measures are undertaken.

Therapy

The broad approach to the treatment of peritonitis is a reflection of the diverse causes and effects.

Early aggressive therapy is required if treatment is to be of benefit, and should be directed at correcting the cause of the peritonitis if possible and overcoming the infection and the effects of inflammation. Support of homeostatic functions includes a repair of fluid, electrolyte, acid–base and protein disturbances, as well as protection of the vital organ systems. Control of contamination is directed at the early removal or closure of the source, including management of external wounds.

Initial introduction of antibiotic coverage directed against the most common pathogens implicated in peritonitis is indicated while awaiting culture results. Peritonitis may be associated with infection by any of the aerobic or anaerobic bacteria found in the intestinal tract. Alternatively, as in the case of abscesses, specific organisms such as *Streptococcus equi*, *Streptococcus zooepidemicus* and *Rhodococcus equi* may be involved. Anaerobic organisms, particularly *Bacteroides fragilis*, which is present in approximately 10 per cent of septic peritonitis cases, may also be implicated. Antimicrobial combinations have been shown to decrease mortality and abscess formation. In one report, 70 per cent of 30 cases of peritonitis were successfully treated with antibiotics and support therapy (Dyson, 1983). However, in a series of 67 cases Hawkins *et al.* (1993) reported a mortality rate of 59.7 per cent.

Procaine penicillin (15 000–20 000 units/kg i/m bid) is suitable as a first choice antibiotic because it is well tolerated, produces peritoneal fluid levels in excess of minimum inhibitory concentration and is bactericidal against most Gram-positive aerobic organisms and most anaerobic organisms. It is not effective against *Bacteroides fragilis*, which should be treated with metronidazole (15 mg/kg *per os* every 6–8 hours). For Gram-negative aerobic organisms and *Rhodococcus equi*, gentamycin (6.6 mg/kg intravenously sid) is recommended. Antimicrobial therapy often needs to be prolonged (> 3 weeks), and the decision to discontinue therapy is based on clinical response and return of WBC count, fibrinogen and peritoneal fluid constituents to normal or near normal levels. In cases where bacteria are susceptible to trimethoprin-sulfadiazine (15–20mg/kg per os bid), this combination provides a useful alternative and has the advantage that the owner can administer these agents for the prolonged period frequently required.

Non-steroid anti-inflammatory drugs should be used to combat toxaemia and provide mild analgesia. Larvicidal anthelmintics such as ivermectin are indicated when parasitism is thought to be the cause of the peritonitis.

Abdominal drainage and lavage

Intermittent drainage of peritoneal fluid is advocated to aid in removal of bacteria, toxins and debris, decrease adhesion formation and pain and increase antimicrobial contact within the peritoneal cavity. The use of peritoneal lavage is controversial, particularly in cases of localized or chronic peritonitis, where there is a risk of disseminating the infection. It may be more beneficial in cases of generalized peritonitis. Two closed system approaches to peritoneal drainage and lavage are possible. Retrograde irrigation through a ventrally placed Foley catheter or thoracic drain, which acts as both an ingress and egress drain, is just as effective and less complicated than placement of ingress drains in both paralumbar fossae for infusion of fluids and a ventral drain for removal of the infused fluids. Large volumes (20–30 l) of Hartmann's solution or lactated Ringer's solution are infused twice a day for several days. Antibiotics added to the fluid do not appear to help, and are best given systemically. Following infusion of the fluid, the drainage tube is clamped and the horse is given a few minutes walking exercise. Two hours later the clamp is removed. The use of a Heimlich valve allows fluid to drain continuously without the risk of aspiration of air.

Premature obstruction of the drain with omentum or fibrin is often a problem, and local tissue irritation and cellulitis resulting from leakage of fluid into the subcutaneous tissues are other complications.

The anatomy and the massive amount of viscera and mesentery make effective lavage difficult to achieve in the horse, and the efficacy of both methods has been questioned. Greater success is achieved if the peritoneal lavage is performed at the time of surgical exploration to identify and correct the underlying cause of the peritonitis.

Prognosis

Prognosis depends on the severity and duration of the peritonitis, the primary underlying cause and the occurrence of complications, including adhesions, abdominal abscesses and organ failure. If the causal lesion can be rapidly identified and corrected, the prognosis is fair to good in localized and mild acute diffuse peritonitis. In chronic cases, or cases complicated by severe abdominal contamination or intestinal perforation, the prognosis is poor.

Anterior (proximal) enteritis

Anterior enteritis is an inflammatory, oedematous and haemorrhagic disease of the proximal small intestine in yearlings and adult horses. There may be a history of dietary change, particularly an increase in the energy content.

Clinical signs

The disease can be diagnosed for certain only at surgery or autopsy, but in most cases the signs are specific enough to allow a clinical diagnosis to be made. The acute clinical syndrome is characterized by sudden onset of acute abdominal pain, ileus, large volumes of foetid, alkaline and sometimes brownish-tinged gastric reflux, tachycardia, dehydration and, sometimes, mild pyrexia. The abdominal pain usually subsides after decompression of the stomach, but the patient remains depressed. Heart rate (70–100 bpm) and respiratory rate (30–60) are elevated, and capillary refill time is extended to 4–6 s. Mucous membranes are congested and injected, and borborygmi are absent on abdominal auscultation.

Rectal examination reveals a relatively empty intestinal tract except for a thickened or slightly distended segment of distal duodenum as it courses over the base of the caecum. Distended loops of proximal jejunum may be palpable. The large colon may be reduced in size and contracted down onto the contents, which are dry and firm secondary to the breakdown in intestinal fluid transport.

Laboratory data

The packed cell volume and total plasma protein values reflect severe dehydration, and may be in excess of 55% and 8.5 g/l respectively. Toxic neutrophils and neutropaenia indicate toxaemia; however, early cases often have a neutrophilia. Serum electrolytes are usually normal; however, mild to moderate hypochloraemia is present in 50 per cent of cases. There may be acidosis or alkalosis, depending on the volume of gastric reflux and the severity of the shock. Abdominocentesis findings tend to be unremarkable unless mural necrosis is advanced. The peritoneal fluid is usually straw-coloured and usually clear or slightly cloudy, but in severe cases has a red discoloration with very high protein, red blood cells and increased neutrophils. The absence of blood staining of the fluid can be of value in differentiating this syndrome from strangulation obstruction of the small intestine.

Gross intestinal lesions

At laparotomy or autopsy, varying lengths of the proximal small intestine are found to be slightly to moderately distended. Rarely is its diameter greater than 7 cm, and the intraluminal pressure is usually less than 10 cmH$_2$O. The wall of the duodenum and proximal jejunum is slightly thickened, but is not as oedematous as infarcted bowel and has red and yellow streaks on its surface. The serosa is mottled with petechial and echymotic haemorrhages, which can involve most of the surface.

In some cases, the lesions may progress to focal necrosis of the intestinal wall. Haemorrhage may be seen in the mesoduodenum and mesojejunum, together with subserosal oedema at the junction of the mesentery and intestine. The rest of the small intestine is flaccid, with a normal pink colour. No external signs are visible on the stomach.

Histology

The histological lesions are confined to the duodenum and proximal jejunum in most cases, but can extend to the stomach and colon. There is submucosal and mucosal oedema, hyperaemia and sloughing of the villous epithelium. In severe cases, there is neutrophilic infiltration and degeneration in the submucosa and haemorrhages in the muscularis and submucosa. The severity of lesions varies between cases.

Aetiology

The aetiology of anterior enteritis is uncertain. *Clostridium perfringens* and mycotoxins are the most frequently incriminating causes. The histological lesion is similar to clostridial enteritis seen in young pigs, but is unlike the recognized clostridial enteritis in the horse, which usually produces lesions in the caecum and large colon. However, *Clostridium perfringens* can consistently be cultivated in large numbers (up to 10^6 CFU/g faeces) from gastric and/or small intestinal contents in cases of anterior enteritis in the UK (Griffiths *et al.*, 1997).

Differential diagnosis

The major condition from which anterior enteritis must be differentiated is small intestinal obstruction, but large intestinal diseases or obstruction, peritonitis and other causes of abdominal pain must be considered. In the UK and other European countries, acute grass sickness is another important differential because of the considerable similarity between the presenting signs in this and anterior enteritis – *viz*, colic and depression, gastric reflux, small intestinal distension, secondary large colon impaction, complete ileus and peritoneal fluid with a raised protein content.

Treatment

In the absence of an identified cause for this condition, the management of anterior enteritis has been directed primarily at aggressive supportive therapy rather than at eliminating a specific aetiological agent. Various methods of treatment have been reported, both conservative and surgical.

The major medical therapeutic objectives are as follows:

1. To maintain adequate decompression of the stomach by repeated nasogastric intubation (every 2 hours) to assist in control of pain and reduce the risk of gastric rupture.
2. To replenish lost fluids and electrolytes by intravenous administration of large volumes of polyionic fluids at initial rates of 10–15 l per hour for a 500 kg horse, later reduced to 2–5 l/hour after hydration is restored. Addition of potassium to the fluids at a rate of 15–20 mmol/l and calcium supplementation is also often indicated.
3. To reduce pain and ameliorate the effects of endotoxaemia by low-dose non-steroidal anti-inflammatory therapy such as flunixine meglumine (0.25 mg/kg i/v every 6–8 hours).
4. Although antimicrobial therapy has been a matter of debate, the possibility of infection with Clostridium spp. merits treatment with procaine penicillin or metronidazole.
5. The resumption of intestinal motility, which may be encouraged by the use of prokinetic drugs.

Approximately 80 per cent of horses with anterior enteritis recover with aggressive medical therapy. However, such therapy is often time-consuming and expensive; many cases require treatment for more than 3–4 days and some for as long as 8–10 days, until repair of the damage to the intestine brings about cessation of transudation of fluid into the lumen.

Surgery is an option that is considered by some as unacceptable because the stress involved could increase the risk of post-operative shock and laminitis; however, this has not been the author's experience. At laparotomy, the characteristic gross lesions of the proximal small intestine are identified and other conditions eliminated by systematic examination of the gastrointestinal tract. The small intestine is gently decompressed by massaging its contents into the caecum. When large volumes of fluid are present, the caecum is evacuated via a small enterotomy incision at its apex. 2 g of metronidazole is administered intravenously as soon as the diagnosis is confirmed, and Hartmann's solution is administered during surgery. Every effort is made to keep the procedure as short as possible, usually about 40 minutes from the first incision to completion of abdominal closure.

Nasogastric intubation is performed on recovery and at 3-hourly intervals until no fluid is obtained on two successive occasions. Metronidazole and low-dose flunixin therapy are continued for 2–3 days. Intravenous Hartmann's solution is administered throughout surgery and during the post-operative period until normal hydration and gut activity are restored.

Ninety-six per cent of horses treated in this way recover. They show a steady fall in heart rate and packed cell volume, returning to normal within 24–72 hours of surgery. Less than 20 per cent have any significant volume of gastric reflux, and in these horses it has ceased 12–24 hours after surgery. Restoration of normal bowel activity is rapid, and horses are discharged 6 days post-operatively. The incidence of post-operative complications is very low.

Surgery should be considered, particularly if there is any reasonable doubt about the initial diagnosis. It overcomes the difficulty in differentiating the condition on clinical signs alone from a physical obstruction of the intestine and from grass sickness in those countries in which the condition occurs. By resorting to surgery without delay, complete decompression of the distended proximal small intestine can be achieved, thus encouraging the return of normal perfusion and peristalsis. As a result of the rapid return of normal gut activity and cardiovascular status, the horses require very little post-operative care and hospitalization, which keeps the cost down for the client.

Colitis

Most cases of acute diarrhoea (acute colitis) in adult horses are associated with substantial inflammatory involvement of the caecum and large colon, which are in turn associated with a myriad of systemic and pathophysiologic events. Passage of excess water in faeces reflects a disruption of normal balance of fluid and electrolyte secretion and absorption in the intestinal tract. The cause of the diarrhoea is rarely known at the time of onset of clinical signs, and the aetiology of individual cases of colitis frequently remains obscure despite vigorous diagnostic efforts. Affected horses show signs of abdominal pain, dehydration and shock. Signs of endotoxaemia frequently accompany or even precede diarrhoea in horses. Severe tissue inflammation can result in loss of mucosal epithelium, leading to chronic malabsorption. Metabolic alterations and malabsorption of volatile fatty acids, which result from excessive production and release of inflammatory mediators, lead to energy deficits and catabolism of body tissues. The diarrhoea may be severe and the clinician's efforts, in the face of a rapid clinical progression of the disease, are directed at modifying inflammatory changes and replacing loss of fluids, electrolytes and plasma proteins. Complications that occur in colitis patients, regardless of aetiology, include overwhelming endotoxaemia, laminitis, immune suppression, susceptibility to super-infection with bacteria or fungi, and colonic infarction.

A number of infectious causes of acute colitis have been described – Salmonella spp., *Clostridium perfringens* and, more recently, *Clostridium difficile* and *Ehrlichia risticii*. Other causes include parasites, peritonitis, excessive non-steroidal anti-inflammation drug therapy, antibiotic administration and heavy metal, plant and cantharidin (blister beetle) toxicosis. Cases of acute enterocolitis in which the cause cannot be identified are frequently classified as idiopathic colitis. Such cases are reported to follow incidents of stress, such as surgery, transport, respiratory disease and exhaustive exercise.

Salmonellosis

Salmonellosis is the most frequently diagnosed infectious cause of diarrhoea in horses. All ages are susceptible, but it is most common in young horses. Stress due to transport, anaesthesia and/or surgery, training and recent dietary changes predispose horses to salmonellosis. Serious outbreaks involving large numbers of horses can occur, and it can be a particular problem in equine hospitals. Large numbers of Salmonella serotypes have been associated with equine colitis. Salmonellae are ubiquitous in the environment, and up to 20 per cent of asymptomatic horses may shed Salmonella spp. transiently in their faeces for several days to weeks. Horses, however, are not considered to be carriers *per se*, since no host-adapted Salmonella species currently affect the horse. In contrast to acutely infected horses, which pass large numbers of highly infective salmonellae in diarrhoeic faeces, the number of organisms passed by asymptomatic shedders is usually low, and these animals do not appear to pose a threat to normal healthy horses. They can, however, be the cause of outbreaks of salmonellosis in hospitals and on breeding farms.

Salmonellosis is typically characterized by an acute colitis resulting in profuse, foetid and sometimes bloodstained watery diarrhoea, and systemic effects of a multitude of inflammatory mediators. However, fever, depression together with abdominal pain and leucopenia (with or without a shift to the left) often precede the onset of diarrhoea. Prompt isolation of horses exhibiting these signs will minimize the risk of spread to other horses on the premises. Proximal enteritis with gastric reflux can occur. Heart and respiratory rates are elevated, and the mucous membranes are injected. Gut sounds may be decreased or absent early in the course of the disease. Severely affected horses have septicaemia and endotoxaemia, and are profoundly dehydrated, hyponatraemic, hypokalaemic and azotaemic. There is an accompanying metabolic acidosis and horses that have had profuse diarrhoea for several days develop marked hypoproteinaemia. Milder forms exist.

The complications that may result from Salmonella septicaemia include laminitis, thrombophlebitis (DIC), hepatitis, nephritis, and chronic colitis resulting in chronic diarrhoea.

Multiple (three to five) faecal cultures on successive days for Salmonella spp. should be performed on all horses with diarrhoea to enhance the likelihood of isolation of the organism. Ideally 5–10 g of formed faeces should be submitted, but samples of watery faeces from horses with profuse diarrhoea will usually yield a positive result on culture.

In many cases of salmonellosis, aggressive treatment facilitates resolution of the severe diarrhoea and associated metabolic disorders within 7–10 days of the onset of illness. However, horses that develop salmonellosis post-colic surgery frequently succumb to the disease. Survival is also unlikely in horses that have had severe diarrhoea and toxaemia for 10 days or longer, since they have extensive loss of colonic mucosa and severe inflammatory changes in the colon wall.

Clostridial colitis

Clostridial diarrhoea has been diagnosed, but confirming the diagnosis is more difficult than for salmonellosis. It is necessary to culture faeces anaerobically, and often in special media. In addition to culture of the organism, isolation of clostridial toxins enhances confirmation of the aetiology of the colitis.

Clostridium perfringens type A has been described as a cause of peracute, toxaemic colitis (colitis x), but it is unclear whether it is an important or infrequent aetiological agent in horses (Murray, 1996). Strains of *Cl. perfringens* type A are classified on the basis of toxins produced, with at least 12 identified to date (Shone and Hambleton, 1988).

Diarrhoea in foals (Jones *et al.*, 1988) and a fatal colitis in mares whose foals were treated with erythromycin and rifampicin for *Rhodococcus equi* pneumonia (Baverud *et al.*, 1997) have been reported associated with *Cl. difficile*.

Cl. difficile produces two toxins, A and B, which have both enterotoxigenic and cytogenic properties (Shone *et al.*, 1988). In addition, toxin A is a potent neutrophilic chemotoxic agent and stimulates cytokine release by macrophages (Pathaulakis *et al.*, 1990). The clinical signs described for clostridiosis vary from peracute haemorrhagic fatal colitis to signs similar to those of colitis caused by Salmonella. Death or euthanasia on the grounds of extreme unresponsive pain may occur prior to diarrhoea. Affected horses are severely toxaemic and show fever, injected mucous membranes, PCV often > 60 per cent and rapid progressive cardiovascular collapse. A suspicion of clostridial diarrhoea is heightened by association with antimicrobial therapy, but diagnosis depends on isolation of pathogenic clostridia and identification of toxins.

Treatment with metronidazole (15 mg/kg three or four times daily) or zinc bacitracin (25–50 g premix *per os* every 12 hours) have been suggested for clostridial diarrhoea.

Potomac horse fever

Potomac horse fever is an infectious enterocolonic disorder, believed to be caused by *Ehrlichia risticii*. This obligate intracellular parasite initially infects monocytes and macrophages. All ages of horse are susceptible, and the condition may occur sporadically or in outbreaks in endemic areas. The association between an infected horse and proximity to a river remains strong. The mode of transmission is not known at the present time, although it does not appear to be horse to horse. An insect vector as well as an intermediate mammalian host may be involved in the transmission of the disease in the field.

The clinical signs and complications are similar to those in horses with salmonellosis. Typically, 2–4 days after infection horses show a mild transient fever, which often goes undetected. By 10–14 days post-infection, the horse will become febrile, have a poor appetite and exhibit mild to severe gastrointestinal signs ranging from mild colic and soft faeces to profuse diarrhoea (Murray, 1996). Horses with Potomac horse fever exhibit signs resembling endotoxaemia, including leucopenia. congested mucous membranes and hypercoagulability, as do horses with salmonellosis. Laminitis is a frequent complication.

Paired acute and convalescent blood samples from suspected cases should be submitted for indirect fluorescent antibody or, preferably, ELISA testing for antibodies to *Ehrlichia risticii*. A four-fold increase is considered to confirm infection, but failure to seroconvert does not rule out infection. Once a horse recovers from the disease the infectious agent appears to be eliminated, and horses do not remain chronic carriers. A few may have clinical relapses, which are responsive to tetracycline administration 2–3 weeks after resolution of the initial clinical signs. Vaccination has appeared to diminish the incidence of the disease, but Potomac horse fever can occur in vaccinated animals, although the severity of the disease is less (Murray, 1996).

Diarrhoea associated with antimicrobial therapy

The onset of acute diarrhoea in the horse has been associated with the use of several antibiotics. Diarrhoea is presumed to be secondary to disruption of normal colonic microflora, leading to proliferation of enteropathogens and abnormal production of volatile fatty acids and disruption of normal secretion/absorption patterns. Salmonella spp. and *Clostridium perfringens* and *Clostridium difficile* have been implicated.

Lincomycin administered orally (Raisbeck *et al.*, 1981) and tetracycline given parenterally (Anderson *et al.*, 1971) have been demonstrated to induce severe diarrhoea in horses. Oral administration of erythromycin, penicillin, metronidazole and trimethoprim sulfa have similarly been associated with diarrhoea and, sometimes, fatal colitis in animals treated with these drugs, though this appears to be limited to individuals rather than being a general problem in all horses.

Other causes of colitis

Excessive non-steroidal anti-inflammatory drug therapy can result in diarrhoea secondary to the development of hypoproteinaemia and caecal and colonic mucosal oedema. Acute diarrhoea in adult horses has also been associated with granulomatous enteritis, intestinal lymphosarcoma, peritonitis, heavy metal toxicosis and stress.

Treatment of acute colitis

In cases of acute colitis, fluid administration remains the treatment of primary importance to replace volume, sodium, chloride and potassium losses. Often large volumes are required for several days. The rate of fluid administration depends on the immediacy of the animal's fluid requirements. In a severely dehydrated horse, fluid can be pumped intravenously at a rate of 1 l/min. Administration of 30 l of polyionic crystalloid solution intravenously in 30 minutes to such a horse will improve intravascular volume tremendously. Bicarbonate must be administered intravenously to horses with a metabolic acidosis. Oral administration of fluid is an effective adjunct to intravenous fluid therapy, and reduces the cost. Although severely ill patients will not usually drink voluntarily, once fluid and electrolyte deficits have been partially corrected horses will consume fluids, often selecting water to which electrolytes have been added rather than fresh water.

In severely dehydrated horses in shock, hypertonic saline (2–3 l of a 7 per cent solution) intravenously to help maintain circulating volume is given while hydration is restored. The solution is valuable in severe cases of colitis or endotoxic shock. Adequate volumes of isotonic solutions to re-establish intracellular and extracellular hydration must follow hypertonic saline administration.

Most horses with colitis become hypoproteinaemic, secondary to protein leakage through inflamed colon and catabolism of albumin secondary to negative energy balance. This frequently leads to oedema in several areas of the body, including the intestine. When plasma proteins are less than 4.0 g/dl, plasma transfusions are beneficial, but 8–10 l intravenously are required for effective replacement. If only commercial plasma is available, the cost is often prohibitive.

The nutritional requirements of the colitis patient must also be borne in mind. Even if the horse eats, it is likely to be in severe calorific deficit for some time.

The problems of the associated endotoxaemia in horses with colitis may be addressed by low-dose administration of flunixin meglumine

(0.25–0.5 mg/kg every 6–8 hours) and the use of cross-reactive antibody produced by immunizing horses to *E. coli* J5 strain lipopolysaccharide, which is now commercially available. Clinical experience suggests that in some cases this treatment is successful in moderating the effects of endotoxaemia, particularly when given early in the course of the illness (Murray, 1997). Dimethyl-sulfoxide (DMSO) at a dose rate of 100–200 mg/kg per day, which scavenges hydroxy radicals produced by metabolically activated neutrophils, may be beneficial during the acute stage of colitis, when there is frequently a pronounced neutrophilic invasion of the caecum and colon.

Whether or not antimicrobials should be used in the treatment of colitis is a matter of controversy. In cases of Potomoc horse fever, tetracycline (6.6–11 mg/kg intravenously once or twice daily) has been reported to be effective both clinically and experimentally against *E. risticii* (Palmer, 1984), and some cases of clostridial colitis respond dramatically if treated with metronidazole very early in the course of the disease. However, in the case of Salmonella colitis, even when specific antimicrobial sensitivities to the Salmonella spp. have been established, administration of antimicrobials such as trimethoprim sulfa, gentamycin or a third generation cephalosporin does not significantly alter the course of the disease nor speed up elimination of the organism from the body (Murray, 1997).

Although medications such as kaolin, activated charcoal and bismuth subsalicylate are sometimes used in adult horses with colitis, their efficacy as antisecretory agents has not been established.

Right dorsal colitis

Right dorsal colitis is a relatively new disease, which has been reported in the United States (Cohen *et al.*, 1995a, 1995b) but not in the United Kingdom. The chief complaint is often non-specific, but signalment and history can provide important information which, in some cases, can allow a presumptive diagnosis of the condition to be made. Most commonly there is a history of anorexia, lethargy and recurrent colic. Depending on the duration of the disease, weight loss may be observed and diarrhoea has been described. A history of administration of non-steroidal anti-inflammatory drugs, especially phenylbutazone, is of particular importance, although treatment is often with smaller doses or for shorter durations than would be considered toxic for this drug (Cohen *et al.*, 1995a, 1995b). Ponies, dehydrated horses and young performance horses may be predisposed.

Clinicopathological abnormalities found in horses with right dorsal colitis include hypocalcaemia, anaemia, hypoproteinaemia and hypo-albuminaemia. The leucocyte count is often normal, but leucocytosis and hyperfibrinogenaemia associated with inflammation, and leucopenia and neutropenia, possibly caused by endotoxaemia, can be seen in some cases.

The pathological changes in the right dorsal colon are similar to those of colonic ulcers and strictures caused by the same class of drugs in human beings. Grossly, the lesion is characterized by multifocal to coalescing ulcerations, with discrete areas of mucosal regeneration. In chronic and severe cases, the colon wall can become fibrotic, leading to stenosis, impaction and even colon rupture (Karcher *et al.*, 1990). Findings on gastroscopy can be normal, but some horses have concurrent gastric ulcers.

Localization of the problem exclusively to the right dorsal colon can only be made anatomically by examining the alimentary tract at laparotomy or during necropsy. Diagnosis is therefore based on history, clinical signs and laboratory findings, although ultrasound examination might be useful to show thickening of the right dorsal colon wall (Cohen *et al.*, 1995a, 1995b).

Although reports of right dorsal colitis in horses have described surgical treatment, the prognosis is poor. Surgical access to the lesion is restricted, but the lesion can be bypassed successfully by side-to-side anastomosis between an accessible part of the right dorsal colon and the proximal small colon. However, in most horses, even those in which the diagnosis is made at surgery, dietary management and discontinuation of non-steroidal anti-inflammatory drugs provide a better option. Dietary management consists of feeding pelleted feed and restricting or eliminating roughage for a period of at least 3 months, to decrease the mechanical and physiologic load on the affected segment of bowel (Cohen *et al.*, 1995a, 1995b). Concentrate should be fed as small, frequent meals. Evidence for specific medical treatment is lacking, but the use of psyllium muciloid (4 g into feed every other day), metronidazole and sucralfate should be considered. Misoprostol, a prostaglandin E_2 analogue, could provide protection to the equine colonic mucosa, but it is possible that undesirable side effects such as abdominal pain and diarrhoea could limit its use in some horses.

Gastrointestinal ulcers

Gastro-duodenal ulcer disease

Gastric ulcers were first reported in the foal as an incidental *post mortem* finding (Rooney, 1964). However, they were not reported as a clinical problem until the early 1980s. Advances in technology have made gastroscopes more widely available, and the clinical disease is now recognized in foals, yearlings and mature horses.

The unique anatomy of the equine stomach probably plays a role in the high incidence of gastric ulcers reported. Unlike that of most species, it has a large non-glandular portion covered by stratified squamous epithelium. The glandular portion is similar to other species, and comprises cardiac, fundic and pyloric regions. The margo plicatus forms the junction between glandular and non-glandular mucosa. The most common location for ulcers is the non-glandular mucosa along the margo plicatus on the lesser curvature. This appears endoscopically to be the most dynamic portion, and it is also the area of non-glandular mucosa exposed to gastric acid. It lacks a mucus/bicarbonate layer, and has minimal resistance to exposure to hydrochloric acid. The majority of ulcers in the glandular region of the equine stomach are associated with the use of non-steroidal anti-inflammatory drugs.

The pathogenesis of gastric ulceration, while not fully understood, is undoubtedly multifactorial, with an imbalance between aggressive and protective factors playing a pivotal role. The principal aggressive factors are hydrochloric acid and pepsin, whereas the protective factors include the mucus/bicarbonate barrier, prostaglandin E_2, mucosal blood flow, cellular restitution and growth factors that promote angiogenesis and mucosal proliferation. Delayed emptying and prolonged gastric contractions are also implicated in the pathogenesis of gastric ulceration. Horses secrete acid even when not eating, and gastric pH can fall below 2.0 soon after they stop eating. Twenty-four hour gastric acidity is significantly less in horses with hay available when compared with that of horses deprived of food. Those turned out to pasture full time have a gastric pH of 5–6.5, and typically have no gastric ulcers. *Helicobacter pylori* is now generally accepted as being the principal cause of peptic ulceration and gastritis in humans, but there is no evidence to date of *H. pylori* or related Helicobacter species infection in horses. Concentrate feeding may contribute to ulceration by increasing serum gastrin levels and, presumably, acid secretion by reducing roughage intake and, most importantly, the time the horse spends eating.

Gastro-duodenal ulcer disease affects foals, yearlings and adult horses, and different clinical syndromes and lesion distribution occur in each group.

Gastric ulcer disease in mature horses

The risk factors for gastric ulcer disease (GUD) in adult horses include fasting, stall confinement and strenuous exercise, all of which result in excessive exposure of the non-glandular portion of the stomach to excessive amounts of acid. Even when hay is fed, there is still great variation in gastric pH throughout the day (Murray, 1996). GUD is rarely seen in horses at pasture. Lesions in the glandular area may be associated with administration of non-steroidal anti-inflammatory drugs and are commonly present in severely ill horses. Horses with delayed gastric emptying or reflux of intestinal contents are also prone to gastric ulcers.

Clinical signs

Few horses with GUD have noticeable clinical signs, and the severity of the lesions does not always correlate with the presence or absence of clinical signs. Affected animals may have a poor appetite and are slower to clear up grain, and some may show weight loss. Depression and occasional pawing of the ground are the most common signs of abdominal pain; severe colic is rare. Small ulcers that bleed are more likely to cause pain. Poor performance is also a common sign in racehorses with gastric ulcers.

Diagnosis

The diagnosis is based on clinical signs and endoscopic examination of the stomach, but a complete physical examination and rapid response to therapy with H_2/proton pump blockers or H_2-antagonists are required to determine if gastric ulcers are responsible for the clinical signs.

To adequately examine the stomach of an adult horse, an endoscope 3 m long is required. Shorter endoscopes of 2–2.2 m will reach the stomach, but will limit the examination to the margo plicatus and not allow visualization of the lesser curvature and pyloric region. To adequately visualize the surface of the stomach, food is withheld for at least 12 hours and water for 6 hours. If some feed material remains on the surface, it may be removed by directing water via the biopsy channel onto the mucosal surface or, preferably, by attaching a roller pump to the biopsy port.

Ulcers within the squamous mucosa may be divided into two categories, acute and chronic, based on the gross and histologic appearance. Endoscopically acute ulcers are characterized by vertical edges and lack of discernible mucosal thickening. In contrast, chronic ulcers are characterized by sloping edges and hyperplasia of the adjacent mucosa. Ulcers may be seen to bleed after inflation of the stomach or removal of adherent food material. Both acute and chronic ulcers may be seen in the same horse, suggesting that, as some ulcers heal, new ones are formed if an inciting cause persists. Observations suggest that naturally occurring ulcers heal within approximately 2 weeks when the horse is turned out to pasture with access to a predominantly hay-based diet (Vasitas *et al.*, 1997). Chronic ulcers generally remain unless the horse is treated with anti-ulcer medication or removed from the environment originally responsible for ulcer development.

Ulcers within the glandular region of the stomach have been reported in 4 per cent of racing thoroughbreds (Vasitas *et al.*, 1984) but are probably less common in the general adult horse population. Glandular ulcers are usually identified by the presence of either acute haemorrhage or brown material formed by blood denatured by gastric acid.

Gastric ulcer disease in foals

Gastric ulceration is highly prevalent in foals and has been reported in up to 50 per cent of foals examined endoscopically (Murray *et al.*, 1987, 1990). Gastric ulceration can occur and resolve with no apparent clinical signs, but can also cause significant clinical problems.

Risk factors comprise any concurrent disease or events causing physiological stress and/or dehydration; for example, a recent episode of diarrhoea (highest risk factors, lameness or pneumonia) and the use of non-steroidal anti-inflammatory drugs. Foals commonly have severe lesions on the lesser curvature (non-glandular portion) of the stomach. In young foals and/or horses, ulcers associated with non-steroidal anti-inflammatory drugs can be equally severe in the glandular area. Duodenal ulceration occurs primarily in older foals, although it is diagnosed in yearlings.

Clinical signs

In contrast to the adult horse, the clinical signs in foals are dramatic and characteristic. The earliest signs are failure to nurse adequately, bruxism, colic and dorsal recumbency. Signs of salivation or oesophageal reflux indicate gastric outflow obstruction or pseudo-obstruction with gastro-oesophageal reflux, reflecting severe ulceration of the pylorus and/or duodenum and, sometimes, oesophagus.

Pale mucous membranes, weight loss and diarrhoea are other clinical signs which may be observed. The most severe signs are associated with gastric duodenal perforation, which can occur in foals with no previous illness. These animals may be found dead or in acute endoxic shock. Foals present with depression colic and a tense abdomen, and those with small perforations in the squamous mucosa near the cardia have shallow, laboured breathing, suggestive of acute respiratory distress. However, auscultation of the chest reveals no abnormal lung sounds. Ultrasonography and abdominocentesis will confirm peritonitis resulting from perforation.

Diagnosis

The clinical signs are most important, and a presumptive diagnosis can usually be made based on the signs mentioned above. Because the classical clinical signs of gastro-duodenal disease usually signify severe disease, endoscopy will allow the veterinarian to determine whether ulcers are present, the location and severity of the lesions and the type and duration of treatment indicated. However, endoscopy may not be needed and consideration should be given to the stress involved with this procedure in young foals. Most gastric ulcers in foals are located in the squamous mucosa, adjacent to the margo plicatus along the greater and lesser curvature, the distribution varying with the age of the foal. Up to 50 per cent of clinically normal foals less than 1 month of age have erosion or mild ulcers adjacent to the margo plicatus along the greater curvature. These usually heal without treatment, and are not associated with clinical signs. Occasionally, squamous epithelial erosions will become extensive and result in clinical signs, most often diarrhoea, but this will resolve within 24 hours of commencing appropriate gastric acid-suppressive treatment (Murray, 1997). In older foals, more severe ulceration of the squamous epithelium is responsible for signs of abdominal discomfort, and this requires aggressive treatment.

Spontaneously healing, mild erosive lesions in the gastric glandular mucosa can be observed in approximately 10 per cent of normal neonates. A small number of foals with duodenal ulceration develop stricture as the ulceration heals.

Treatment

Successful treatment of gastric ulcers may be achieved by addressing the underlying cause and treating with medications that create an environment conducive to ulcer healing. Decisions concerning whether or not to treat gastric ulcers, what medication to use and for how long are best made on the endoscopic findings. If gastroscopy is unavailable the efficacy of any treatment will have to be judged on clinical signs alone, which are often vague and non-specific.

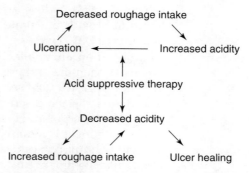

Figure 4.1 Gastric ulcer pathophysiology and healing (Murray, 1996).

Acid-suppressive treatment is often required to break the cycle of inappetance, which causes lowering of gastric pH, which results in ulceration, which then prolongs and exacerbates the inappetance (Fig. 4.1). A significant improvement in the clinical signs, such as poor appetite, colic or diarrhoea (foals), resulting from gastric ulcers is usually seen within 24–48 hours of commencing such treatment. A variety of therapeutic agents are used to treat gastric and/or duodenal ulcers in adult horses and foals (Table 4.4).

H_2 antagonists

Gastric acid secretion can largely be attenuated by the use of histamine receptor-2 (H_2) antagonists. However, although there is ample evidence that they have a significant effect on intragastric pH in fasted horses, scientific evidence that these compounds enhance ulcer healing is lacking.

Cimetidine and ranitidine are the most frequently used H_2 antagonists in the horse. Many dosages have been recommended and, because these drugs are expensive, there is pressure to use as little as possible. However, as the dose of acid suppressive agent is lowered, the percentage of patients that will respond poorly or not at all increases

Table 4.4 Gastric ulcer disease therapy – recommended doses (after MacAllister, 1997)

	mg/kg	*Dosing interval*	*Route*
Cimetidine	20–25	6–8 hrs	PO
Cimetidine	4–6	6–8 hrs	iv, im
Famotidine	1.5–2.5	6–8 hrs	PO
Fenbendazole	10	once daily	PO
Omeprazole	1.0–4.0	once daily	PO
Omeprazole	0.5	once daily	iv
Ranitidine	6–8	6–8 hrs	PO
Ranitidine	1.5–2.0	6–8 hrs	iv, im
Sucralfate	22–30	6 hrs	PO

(Murray, 1996). A dose of 6.6 mg/kg administered orally tid has been found to provide adequate suppression of gastric acidity in the greatest percentage of horses. Although formulations for intravenous administration are available, they are approximately three times more expensive than the oral preparations. Famotidine is a much more potent inhibitor of gastric acid secretion than cimetidine or ranitidine; however, considering the increased cost of famotidine, there is no advantage in using the more potent antagonist. In most horses with gastric ulcers, 3 weeks' treatment is required to ensure complete healing. Whereas 80–90 per cent of adult horses treated with ranitidine at 6.6 mg/kg per os for 3 weeks had complete healing of ulcers, at 2 weeks, complete healing occurred in only 15–40 per cent (Murray, 1996).

Proton pump inhibitors

Blocking of the hydrogen–potassium ATPase proton pump of the apical membrane of the parietal cell causes profound inhibition of gastric acid secretion, regardless of the stimulus.

Omeprazole, the most commonly administered proton pump inhibitor, has a prolonged antisecretory effect, allowing once daily treatment, which is much more convenient than the multiple daily doses required for other anti-ulcer compounds. In a recent vehicle-controlled study (Murray *et al.*, 1997), 17 thoroughbred racehorses with moderately to severe gastric ulceration were administered omeprazole (1.5 mg/kg bwt/day) or vehicle by nasogastric tube once daily. The horses were treated daily until there was no apparent epithelial defect, assessed by thorough endoscopic examination every third or fourth day. The results showed that omeprazole resulted in more rapid and complete gastric ulcer healing (10–21 days) than treatment with vehicle (14–28 days). The fact that spontaneous ulcer healing was observed in vehicle-treated horses underlines the multifactorial nature of ulcer healing, and reflects that suppression of gastric acidity creates a favourable environment within the stomach that promotes healing (Murray *et al.*, 1997).

Omeprazole is currently available in a delayed release capsule, which is marketed for human beings. These capsules can be administered orally in syrup or molasses to horses. It must be borne in mind, however, that it may take 3–5 days to have full effect on gastric acid suppression. Acutely symptomatic or painful horses/foals may require an initial parenteral dose of omeprazole or an H_2 receptor antagonist for a more rapid effect.

Sucralfate

At a pH of 4, sucralfate forms a sticky, viscid gel which adheres to epithelial cells and the base of ulcer craters, where it will remain for more than 6 hours (Brunton, 1990). This coating creates an acid-resistant layer, and protects the ulcer from the effects of gastric acid and pepsin. The beneficial effects include inhibition of pepsin activity, an increase in thickness and quality of the mucus layer, and prevention of mucus degradation.

Although initial studies indicated that a pH of less than 4.0 in the stomach was important for the gel to form, subsequent studies have shown that most of the benefits of sucralfate are not dependent on gastric pH. Its effect appears only to be beneficial in glandular ulceration.

Antacids

Most antacids are mixtures of magnesium hydroxide and aluminium hydroxide. There is no scientific data available on the effects of antacids on gastric ulcer healing in horses. A study on the ability of antacids to raise the gastric pH (Clark and Merritt, 1994) indicated that, in the clinical situation, it would be difficult to administer them in high enough doses or frequently enough to have a long-term clinical effect.

The high cost of anti-ulcer drugs raises the question whether they should be administered to asymptomatic horses with endoscopically confirmed ulcers. The decision as to which cases should be treated should be based on the endoscopic severity of the lesions, the presence and severity of clinical signs, and the value of the horse. Clinical signs usually disappear before complete healing has occurred. For those clinical cases with ulcers that remain severe after 2 weeks of therapy, an additional 2 weeks of treatment is usually recommended (MacAllister, 1997). Most horses will be healed or almost completely healed after 28 days of treatment. If medical therapy is ineffective, or sequelae of duodenal ulceration cause complications, surgical intervention may be required.

Gastroenterostomy has been reported to be effective in some cases to bypass the affected portion of duodenum and allow for gastric emptying. However, the reported survival rates are poor. In addition, these horses require weeks to months of treatment with acid-suppressive drugs and prokinetic drugs until normal gastric emptying is restored.

References

Allen, D. (1985). Small intestinal obstruction: pathophysiology, surgical therapy and post-operative treatment. *Proc. Vet. Sem. Equine Acute Abdomen, University of Georgia,* **1,** 47–9.

Anderson, G., Ekman, L., Mansson, I. *et al.* (1971). Lethal complications following administration of oxytetracycline in the horse. *Nord. Vet. Med.,* **23,** 9–22.

Baverud, V., Franken, A., Gunnarsson, A. *et al.* (1997). *Clostridium difficule* associated with acute colitis in mares when their foals are treated with erythromycin and refampicin for *Rhodococcus equi.* Abstracts from *Gastroenterologi hos häst. Nodiskt hästpraktikermöte, Skara, Sweden,* 2–3 October, pp. 55.

Boening, K. J. and von Saldern, F. C. H. (1986). Non-surgical treatment of left dorsal displacement of the large colon of horses under general anaesthesia. *Proc. of the Equine Colic Res. Symp., Athens, Georgia,* p. 325. University of Georgia.

Brunton, L. L. (1990). Drugs affecting gastrointestinal function. In *The Pharmacologic Basis of Therapeutics,* pp. 897–913. Goodman and Gillmans.

Clark, C. K. and Merritt, A. M. (1994). Effect of Maalox TC or bismuth subsalicylate on gastric pH in fed horses. *Proc. 40th Ann. Conv. Am. Assoc. Equine Pract.,* p. 127.

Cohen, N. D., Carter, G. K., Mealey, R. H. *et al.* (1995). Medical management of right dorsal colitis in five horses. A retrospective study (1987–1993). *J. Vet. Intern. Med.,* **9,** 272.

Cohen, N. D., Mealer, R. A., Chaffin, M. K. *et al.* (1995). The recognition and medical management of right dorsal colitis in horses. *Vet. Med.,* **90,** 687.

Dyson, S. (1983). Review of 30 cases of peritonitis in the horse. *Equine Vet. J.*, **15,** 25–30.

Edwards, G. B. (1997). Diseases and surgery of the small colon. *Vet. Clin. N. Am. Equine Pract.*, **13(2),** 359.

Embertson, R. M. (1997). Colopexy to prevent recurrent large colon volvulus or displacement. *Proc. 5th Cong. Equine Med. Surg., Geneva,* 14th–16th Dec., p. 134.

Embertson, R. M., Colahan, P. T., Brown, M. P. *et al.* (1985). Ileal impaction in the horse. *J. Am. Vet. Med. Assoc.*, **186,** 570.

Fischer, A. T. and Meagher, D. M. (1986). Strangulating torsion of the equine large colon. *Comp. Cont. Educ. Pract. Vet.*, **8,** 525–30.

Freeman, D. (1997). Surgery of the small intestine. *Vet. Clin. N. Am. Equine Pract.*, **13(2),** 262.

Griffiths, N. J., Walton, J. R. and Edwards, G. B. (1997). An investigation of the prevalence of the toxigenic types of *Clostridium perfringens* in horses with anterior enteritis. Preliminary results. *Aerobe,* **3,** 121–5.

Hardy, J., Bedwarski, R. M. and Biller, D. S. (1994). Effect of phenylephrine on haemodynamics and splenic dimensions in horses. *Am. J. Vet. Res.*, **55,** 1570.

Hawkins, J. F., Bowman, K. F., Roberts, M. C. and Cowe, P. (1993). Peritonitis in horses: 67 cases (1985–1990). *J. Am. Vet. Med. Assoc.*, **203,** 284–8.

Huskamp, B. (1982). The diagnosis and treatment of acute abdominal conditions in the horse. The various types and frequency as seen at the animal hospital in Hochmoor. *Proc. Equine Colic Res. Symp., University of Georgia,* pp. 261–72.

Huskamp, B. (1998a). Incarcerated inguinal hernia; diagnosis and treatment. *Int. Sem: Update on Equine Colic, Bologna,* 2nd May, pp. 56–62.

Huskamp, B. (1998b). Chronic recurrent caecal impaction: diagnosis, treatment and long-term results. *Int. Sem: Update on Equine Colic, Bologna,* 2nd May, pp. 135–9.

Johnston, J. K. (1996). The use of phenylophrine in the treatment of large colon displacement in the horse. *Vet. Surg.*, **25,** 13.

Jones, R. L., Shidelar, R. K. and Cockerill, G. L. (1988). Association of *Clostridium difficile* with foal diarrhoea. *Proc. 5th Int. Conf. Equine Infect. Dis.*, pp. 236–40.

Kalsbeek, H. C. (1989). Further experiences with non-surgical correction of nephrosplenic entrapment of the left colon in the horse. *Equine Vet. J.*, **21,** 442.

Karcher, L. F., Dill, S. G., Anderson, W. I. *et al.* (1990). Right dorsal colitis. *J. Vet. Intern. Med.*, **4,** 247.

MacAllister, C. G. (1997). Therapy for equine gastric ulcers. *Proc. 5th Cong. Equine Med. Surg., Geneva,* 14th–16th December, pp. 104–8.

Meagher, D. M. (1974). Surgery of the large intestine in the horse. *Arch. Am. Coll. Vet. Surg.*, **3,** 9.

Murray, M. J. (1996). Disorders of the stomach and disorders of the large intestine. *In Large Animal Internal Medicine* (B. P. Smith, ed.), 2nd edn, pp. 710–19 and 723–30. Mosby.

Murray, M. J., Hart, J. and Parker, G. A. (1987). Equine gastric ulcer syndrome. Prevalence of gastric lesions in asymptomatic foals. *Proc. Am. Assoc. Equine Pract., New Orleans,* p. 769.

Murray, M. J., Murray, C. M., Sweeney, H. J. *et al.* (1990). The prevalence of gastric ulcers in foals in Ireland and England. An endoscopic survey. *Equine Vet. J.*, **22,** 6.

Murray, M. J., Haven, M. L., Eichorn, E. S. *et al.* (1997). Effects of omeprazole on healing of naturally occurring gastric ulcers in thoroughbred racehorses. *Equine Vet. J.*, **29(6),** 425–9.

Murray, M. J. (1997). Gastro-duodenal ulceration and acute colitis. *Curr. Ther. Equine Med.*, **4,** 191–203.

von Plocki, K. (1995). Abdominal inguinal herniotomy – a new method of surgical treatment of inguinal hernia/scrotal hernia in the horse. *Proc. 4th ECVS Meeting, Constance, Germany,* pp. 94–5.

Palmer, J. E. (1992). Ptomac horse fever. In *Current Therapy in Equine Medicine* (N. E. Robinson, ed.), pp. 250–53. W. B. Saunders.

Pathaulakis, C., Becker, S. D. and La Mont, J. T. (1990). Mechanism of action of *Cl. difficile* toxins. In *Cl. Difficile-associated Intestinal Diseases* (J.-C. Rambaud and R. Ducluzeau, eds), pp. 55–61. Springer-Verlag.

Ragle, C. A., Meagher, D. M., Schroder, D. L. *et al.* (1989). Abdominal auscultation in the detection of experimentally-induced gastrointestinal sand accumulation. *J. Int. Med.*, **3,** 12.

Raisbeck, M. F., Holt, G. R. and Osweiler, G. D. (1981). Lincamycin-associated colitis in horses. *J. Am. Vet. Med. Assoc.*, **179,** 362–3.

Rooney, J. R. (1964). Gastric ulceration in foals. *Pathologia Vet.*, **1,** 497–503.

Rose, J. A. and Rose, E. M. (1987). Colonic obstruction in the horse: Radiographic and surgical considerations. *Proc AAEP Ann. Conv.*, pp. 95–102.

Ruggles, A. J. and Ross, M. W. (1991). Medical and surgical management of small colon impaction in horses: 28 cases. *J. Am. Vet. Med. Assoc.*, **199,** 1702.

Shone, C. C. and Hambleton, P. (1988). Toxigenic clostridia. In *Biotechnology Handbooks: Clostridia* (N. P. Monton and D. J. Clark, eds), pp. 265–92. Plenum Press.

Sivula, N. J. (1990). Displacement of the large colon associated with non-surgical correction of large colon entrapment in the renosplenic space in a mare. *J. Am. Vet. Med. Assoc.*, **197,** 1190.

Snyder, J. R., Pascoe, J. R., Olander, H. J. *et al.* (1990). Intra-operative assessment of equine colonic tissue for determining viability (abstract). *Vet. Surg.*, **19,** 76.

Vasitas, N. J., Snyder, J. R. and Johnson, B. (1997). Adult stomach and duodenum. In *Equine Endoscopy* (J. L. Traub-Dargatz and C. M. Brown, eds), 2nd edn, pp. 172–86. Mosby, St. Louis.

Vasitas, N. J., Carlson, G. P., Johnson, B. *et al.* (1994). Gastric ulceration in racing thoroughbreds: A pathologic and epidemiologic study. *Gastroenterology*, **106(4),** 848.

White, N. A. (1985). Risk and prognosis of the equine patient with colic. *Proc. Vet. Sem. Equine Acute Abdomen, Georgia*, **1,** 50–51.

White, N. A. and Dabareiner, R. M. (1997). Treatment of impaction colics. *Vet. Clin. N. Am. Equine Pract.*, **13(2),** 254.

White, N. A. (1990). Epidemiology and etiology of equine colic. In *The Equine Acute Abdomen* (N. A. White, ed.), pp. 49–64. Lea and Febiger.

5 Prognosticating the equine acute abdomen

Introduction

Prognosticating the individual case of equine colic can be difficult. The signs that occur during an acute abdomen can vary widely, even for the same disease, making prediction of the outcome an inaccurate science. There is no sign or group of clinical values that can accurately predict the survival of a horse with colic 100 per cent of the time. However, the reality of economic decisions made by horse owners makes the prognosis an important part of the veterinarian's plan for treatment. The cost of treating the horse with a serious intestinal disease can be high, particularly in light of the high complication rate of some diseases. Therefore, the prognosis may be the deciding factor in the type of treatment or in whether a horse is treated at all.

Making an accurate prediction about survival is only a problem in relatively few cases in the normal horse population or typical ambulatory practice, since most horses with colic survive. Most studies have used positive predictive or negative predictive values to help determine the usefulness of specific tests in predicting survival. However, when the prevalence of death is low, test results applied to individual cases will result in less accurate predictions. Therefore, when attempting to give odds of survival, clinical experience must be combined with other predictive values to avoid false positive or negative results.

Chances of immediate survival

The chief question posed when colic is severe is, 'what is the prognosis for life?'. Some clinical signs can be correlated with the chances of survival. Those signs that reflect the cardiovascular response are the best indicators of survival, as they measure the degree of shock (Bristol, 1982; Byars and Thorpe, 1982; Donawick et al., 1977; Furr et al., 1994; Hunt et al., 1986; Gosset et al., 1987; Johnstone and Crane, 1986; Moore et al., 1976; Orsini et al., 1988; Parry et al., 1983a, 1983b; Parry, 1986; Puotenen-Reinert, 1986; Reeves et al., 1986; Reeves et al., 1987; White and Lessard, 1986). Other signs are hard to quantify, but are still related to the chance of survival. These include the degree of pain or depression, the frequency of pain and the ability to control it, the degree of distension of the abdomen, or of the intestine found on rectal exam, mucous membrane colour and abdominal borborygmi (Adams and McIlwraith, 1978; Parry et al., 1983; Puotenen-Reinert, 1986).

Pain, when described as slight, periodic, continuous or violent, and lethargy, were indicative of survival rates of 92, 76, 69, 42 and 25 per cent respectively (Puotenen-Reinert, 1986). Continuous pain increased the chance of death by five times, and uncontrollable pain by 16 times, when compared to horses with a history of colic but with no pain at the time of examination (Reeves *et al.*, 1987). Similarly, horses with a distended intestine on examination *per rectum* were 2.5 times more likely to die than if the bowel palpated was normal, and 3.5 times more likely to die if the distension was in the small intestine (Reeves *et al.*, 1987). Lack of intestinal sound compared to normal sounds in horses with colic increased the risk of dying by 12.7 times. Mucous membrane colour was significantly associated with the risk of dying, horses with red membranes being 8.4 times as likely to die and those with cyanotic membranes 38.2 times more likely to die than horses with normal mucous membranes (Reeves *et al.*, 1987).

Severity of shock

Blood and serum values that accurately measure the severity of shock include the blood pressure, heart rate, PCV, glucose, lactate, BUN, Plt, fibrinogen degradation products(FDP), antithrombin III, prothrombin time, partial thromboplastin time and anion gap (Bristol, 1982; Byars and Thorpe, 1982; Donawick *et al.*, 1977; Furr *et al.*, 1994; Hunt *et al.*, 1986; Gosset *et al.*, 1987; Johnstone and Crane, 1986; Moore *et al.*, 1976; Parry *et al.*, 1983b; Parry, 1986, 1987; Puotenen-Reinert, 1986; Reeves *et al.*, 1986, 1987). Some other quantitative measurements are the peritoneal total protein and the intraluminal hydrostatic pressure of the intestine, which measures the injury to the intestine rather than the cardiovascular status of the horse (Allen *et al.*, 1986). When small intestinal pressures were measured in viable segments at surgery, pressures greater than $15\ cmH_2O$ were associated with a poor chance of survival. Similar predictions have been made by measuring large colon intraluminal pressures at surgery (Moore *et al.*, 1994). Pressures in non-strangulating disease of the large colon varied from $6-46\ cmH_2O$, with all patients surviving. Pressures in strangulating disease ranged from $34-80\ cmH_2O$ in non-survivors and from $4-45\ cmH_2O$ in survivors, with $38\ cmH_2O$ being the most accurate cut-off point for predicting survival.

Presently, the most accurate quantitative measurements that can assist in predicting the chance of survival are those of the severity of dehydration and shock. Systolic blood pressure taken using doppler ultrasound off the coccygeal artery was related to survival (Parry *et al.*, 1983a). Systolic pressures of 50, 80, 110 and 140 mmHg corresponded with probable survival rates of 5, 24, 69 and 94 per cent respectively (Parry, 1986). Heart rates of 40, 80, 100 and 120 bpm have been related to probable survival rates of 90, 50, 25 and 10 per cent respectively (Parry *et al.*, 1983b; Parry, 1986). The PCV has also been found to be helpful, but not as accurate as other values. PCV values of 30, 45, 60 and 65 per cent were associated with probable survival rates of 93, 64, 20 and 10 per cent respectively (Parry, 1986). Lactate values of < 75 mg/dl were associated with a 90 per cent survival (Moore *et al.*, 1976), but the chances of survival declined precipitously to 33 per cent when lactate values were between 75 and 100 mg/dl, and to < 25 per cent at levels greater than 100 mg/dl (Moore *et al.*, 1976). Another report gave no chance of survival with lactate values greater than 100 mg/dl (Donawick *et al.*, 1977).

The anion gap has a similar relationship to the lactate, representing about 82 per cent of the anion gap measured (Gosset *et al.*, 1987). Anion gap is calculated by the following formula:

$$\text{ANIONGAP} = [\text{NA}^+ \text{meq/l}] - [\text{Cl}^- \text{meq/l}] + [\text{HCO}_3^- \text{meq/l}]$$

This can be used to predict survival in cases of colic. In one report, an anion gap of < 20 was associated with a survival of 81 per cent, while a gap of between 20 and 25 gave survival of 47 per cent and a gap of > 25 was associated with a survival of 0 per cent (Bristol, 1982). These measurements appear accurate except in cases of enteritis with low serum chloride values; these horses frequently have a high anion gap but not as high a death rate as predicted.

Glucose has been recognized as an indicator of severe shock. Values greater than 300 mg/dl are associated with high mortality (Parry, 1986). The level of protein in the peritoneal fluid is also related to the survival rate, but is not as good a predictor as some of the other values because of the variability that exists with different diseases. Measurements of total protein in the peritoneal fluid greater than 4.5 g/dl in small intestinal obstruction or strangulation and 3.5 g/dl in large colon obstruction or strangulation indicate a poor prognosis (Allen *et al.*, 1986; White and Lessard, 1986). Though all these results are helpful, there is no way of using individual tests as predictors in individual cases. Only a few of the tests have undergone scrutiny in the form of prospective testing to validate accuracy.

Methods of predicting survival

Parry's multivariate analysis

Parry has provided a method of predicting survival using multivariable analysis, which combines the information of several individual variables simultaneously (Parry *et al.*, 1983b; Parry, 1986). The technique involves calculating a survival index and death index. If the survivor index (SI) value is higher than the death index (DI) value, the horse will most likely survive; however, if the DI is higher than the SI, the horse is more likely to die. The following table gives the equations for the respective survival and death indices (Parry, 1986):

	Survivor index	Death index
Systolic BP	0.125(S) – 8.94	0.0572(S) – 2.44
Lactate	0.0829(L) – 1.40	0.186(L) – 4.26
Bun	0.0993(BUN) – 1.99	0.177(BUN) – 4.83
PCV	0.422(PCV) – 9.73	0.540(PCV) – 15.5

By far the most accurate assessment was provided by the combined formula for the SI:

$$SI = (0.180(S) + 0.213(L) + 0.164(BUN) + 0.486(PCV) - 27.0)$$

compared with the combined formula for the DI:

$$DI = (0.132(S) + 0.330(L) + 0.266(BUN) + 0.582(PCV) - 31.7)$$

This resulted in a combined accuracy of 93 per cent (assuming optimal treatment). Several other models of survival or death probability using logistic regression have been reported (Orsini *et al.*, 1988; Puotenen-Reinert, 1986; Reeves *et al.*, 1986, 1987, 1990), and these formulae provide a prognostic index which helps to predict the likely outcome of the case, assuming optimal treatment.

Colic chart score

In an attempt to make a rapidly usable method of predicting the outcome in colic patients, a Colic Chart Score has been devised by testing 33 common physical or laboratory tests to see which tests, used singly or in combination, give the best prediction of survival (Furr *et al.*, 1994). Cut score values from pulse rate, peritoneal total protein, lactate and mucous membrane refill or colour were placed in groups and assigned scores in a chart (Table 5.1). Measurements are taken from the horse, and the scores assigned are added along the bottom to give a total. Analysis of the scores from a group of horses with colic determined that a total score of 7 or below meant the horse would live, and a score of 8 or above meant the horse would die. When the Colic Chart Score was tested on a new group of horses using the cut score of 8, it accurately predicted death in 100 per cent of the cases. Though this method requires obtaining a lactate value and peritoneal protein, it accurately predicts the outcome in the type of case selected for referral for treatment or surgery. Since lactate values can now be measured by portable machines, it appears that this type of scoring system may eventually be a practical test for field use.

Colic profile

An alternative to calculating the formula is to use the Colic Profile, developed from a project supported by the Morris Animal Foundation (Reeves *et al.*, 1990). This is based on a large number of cases, and provides a formula using easily obtained clinical signs, including evidence of external trauma, heart rate, PCV, selection of medical or surgical treatment and capillary refill time. The formula is particularly

Table 5.1 Colic Chart Score (Furr *et al.*, 1994)

Assigned value	0	1	2	3	4
Pulse (bpm)	< 49	50–60	65–74	75–89	> 90
Peritoneal total protein (g/dl)	< 2.5		2.6–4.0	4.1–4.6	> 4.7
Lactate (mg/dl)	< 49		50–70	80–90	> 90
Mucous membrane	Normal		CRT > 3 or cyanotic		

Total _____ + _____ + _____ + _____ = _____
Colic score < 7, predicted to survive; 8 or >8, predicted to die

suited to use in practice, as it requires easily obtainable information. However, it requires a spreadsheet or programmable calculator to derive the likelihood of death. The prevalence of disease in the population affects the performance of such equations in predicting the prognosis in acute abdominal disease. Where the prevalence of death is low, the formula will be more accurate in predicting which cases will survive. Conversely, if the fatality rate is high, the chances of predicting which cases will die are improved (Reeves *et al.*, 1987). Therefore, when combining the error in predicting survival and non-survival, the totally correct prediction or accuracy ranges between 76 and 82 per cent (Orsini *et al.*, 1988; Reeves *et al.*, 1987; White and Lessard, 1986). These are important numbers to keep in mind, because they show that the possibility of error exists with every prediction.

Scoring chart for prognostication

Because methods for prediction frequently require haematologic or serum values, which are not often available in the field during patient evaluation, a chart has been devised to help categorize the prediction by using clinical signs (Table 5.2). This is not as accurate as measuring specific quantitative values, such as lactate or systolic blood pressure, or using a formula that has been tested on a large number of cases. The chart is a subjective scoring, which uses information from retrospective studies (Orsini *et al.*, 1988; Parry *et al.*, 1983a; Parry, 1986; Puotenen-Reinert, 1986; Reeves *et al.*, 1987, 1990; White and Lessard, 1986). The prognostication is assessed as one of three categories of survival: good (> 90 per cent), guarded (about 50 per cent) and poor (< 25 per cent), and the accuracy cannot be any better than this when using these unweighted and often variable values. It is therefore used only as a guideline, because of the error inherent due to decisions by individual clinicians. The middle zone in this chart is the area of the greatest error; therefore, the chance of survival is going to be given as more than or less than 50 per cent. When giving the odds of survival to the owner, this may be the only fair prediction for horses with these signs. Part of the evaluation will no doubt be subjective, and will have to include historical data. Using one of these values alone has been shown to be inaccurate. Also, when the value of one of the signs does not fit into the same category as the other values, the accuracy of the prognosis will be less. In cases where determining the

Table 5.2 Scoring chart for prognosticating equine acute abdominal cases using physical signs

Prognosis	Good	Guarded	Poor
Heart rate (bpm)	40–59	60–100	> 100
Mucous membrane colour	Pink	Red	Cyanotic
Mucous membrane refill time(s)	1–2	3–4	> 4
PCV (%)	35–45	45–65	> 65
Peritoneal total protein (g/dl)	< 2.5	2.5–4.5	> 4.5

prognosis is an important economic factor, the use of laboratory tests and the above equations or scores is preferred in order to give the highest accuracy in the prognosis.

Summary

The values and methods provided here are helpful in determining a prognosis. However, the veterinarian must remember that the prognosis may change rapidly from good to poor over time, due to the events that occur during progression of intestinal disease. Therefore, to give a good prognosis based on a low lactate or anion gap in a horse that has just entered a violently painful stage is using poor judgement. The prognosis may change rapidly during the time required for transport, treatment, or surgery, and can also change if proper therapy is not provided. On the other hand, a guarded or poor prognosis must be tempered with an observed response to treatment. A horse with no intestinal sounds, an increased heart rate and a high PCV, indicating a poor prognosis, may respond to appropriate treatment. When the physical signs change, including return of borborygmi, a decreasing PCV and a lowered heart rate, a new evaluation to determine a prognosis is indicated. Depending on the case, it is often prudent to see the effects of treatment prior to predicting the outcome. Certainly, both these examples have reasons for caution when giving a prognosis. The study of prognosticating colic has not yet taken these factors into consideration.

Prognosis for short- and long-term survival

There has been little research into determining the long-term survival of a horse following a colic episode, except in cases of surgical colic and impactions (Dabareiner and White, 1995; Ducharme *et al.*, 1983; MacDonald *et al.*, 1989; McCarthy and Hutchins, 1988; Parry, 1987). Mild idiopathic colic does not appear to put the horse at increased risk of death after the colic episode, though no study has been done to define this risk. The risk of death after impaction colic also appears low, with short- and long-term survival in medical cases being equal (95 per cent); however, the long-term survival for impactions treated surgically was lower (57.8 per cent) (Dabareiner and White, 1995). After large colon impaction, horses had a higher frequency of repeat colic than expected in the normal population, and a high case fatality rate in repeat cases in which the horse required surgery (Dabareinter and White, 1995).

There is an increased risk of colic and death after surgery for acute abdominal disease. Short-term survival for surgical disease varies between 35 and approximately 80 per cent, depending on the type of case load and the response and travel time required after recognition (Adams and McIlwraith, 1978; Hunt *et al.*, 1986; MacDonald *et al.*, 1989; McCarthy and Hutchins, 1988; Parker *et al.*, 1989; Philips and Walmsley, 1993). In two studies, short-term survival from general surgical cases at the time of discharge from the hospital is higher than long-term survival of a year or more: 62.8 per cent vs. 45.5 per cent (Ducharme *et al.*, 1983) and 72.2 per cent vs. 66.2 per cent (Philips, 1993). It appears that long-term survival rates may have improved over the 10 years between the two studies, probably due to case selection and improvement in overall case management. Survival after small intestinal resection and anastomosis is much lower due to complications, the most common being adhesions and repeat colic cases (MacDonald *et al.*, 1989). Though there are no studies that give risk factors for complications, it appears that horses in shock or those that develop ileus are more likely to have life-threatening complications, including repeat colic, laminitis, enteritis, peritonitis, diarrhoea, intestinal adhesions and abdominal hernia (Hunt *et al.*, 1986). Further work in this area is needed to help identify cases at high risk of lethal complications.

A greater challenge is in determining whether the disease causing the colic episode will occur again, and there is no magic or scientific way to make this prediction. Some horses are prone to recurrent colic, some at specific times of the year every year, and some erratically. These horses will have colic when other horses in the same environment have no abdominal problems. Also, horses with this type of history may have recurrent colic with no apparent medical reason. One disease complex known to predispose horses to repeat episodes including surgery is the large colon displacement or volvulus, seen most often in the brood mare during late pregnancy or lactation (Philips and Walmsley, 1993). Mares having colic episodes during this time should be considered at risk in future years for colon obstruction or strangulation during the same risk periods. Small intestinal diseases requiring surgery also increase the risk of repeat colic due to adhesions. This complication can cause recurrence for years, but most problems with adhesions are encountered during the first 6 months after surgery.

If the treatment, even with surgery, is successful, the prognosis for future use is usually good (> 90 per cent). Horses have been able to return to all types of activity, including racing, jumping, showing and breeding. Two major complications that can limit a horse's return to its previous activity are abdominal hernia after surgery and laminitis with distal phalanx rotation. Both of these can be life threatening, or can reduce the level of athletic endeavour.

References

Adams, S. B. and McIlwraith, C. W. (1978). Abdominal crisis in the horse: A comparison of pre-surgical evaluation with surgical findings and results. *Vet. Surg.*, **7**, 63–9.

Allen, D., White, N. A. and Tyler, D. E. (1986). Factors for prognostic use in equine obstructive small intestinal disease. *J. Am. Vet. Med. Assoc.*, **189(7)**, 777–80.

Bristol, D. G. (1982). The anion gap as a prognostic indicator in horses with abdominal pain. *J. Am. Vet. Med. Assoc.*, **181**, 63–5.

Byars, T. D. and Thorpe, P. E. (1982). Prognostic significance of fibrin/fibrinogen degradation products in the surgical equine abdominal crisis. *Proc. Equine Colic Res. Symp., Georgia, Athens*, pp. 142–6. University of Georgia.

Dabareiner, R. M. and White, N. A. (1995). Large colon impaction in horses: 147 cases (1985–1991). *J. Am. Vet. Med. Assoc.*, **206**, 679–85.

Donawick, W. J., Ramberg, C. F. and Smith, D. F. (1977). Diagnostic and prognostic values of blood lactate in colic. *Proc. Am. Assoc. Equine Pract. Ann. Conven.*, pp. 247–8.

Ducharme, N. G., Hackett, R. P. and Ducharme, G. R. (1983). Surgical treatment of colic: Results in 181 horses. *Vet. Surg.*, **12**, 206–9.

Furr, M. O., Lessard, P. and White, N. A. (1994). The use of a Colic Chart Score to predict the outcome of acute abdominal disease in the horse. *Vet. Surg.*, **24**, 97–101.

Hunt, J. M., Edwards, G. B. and Clarke, K. W. (1986). Incidence, diagnosis and treatment of post-operative complications in colic cases. *Equine Vet. J.*, **18**, 264–70.

Gosset, K. A., Cleghorn, B., Martin, G. S. and Church, G. E. (1987). Correlation between anion gap, blood lactate concentration and survival in horses. *Equine Vet. J.*, **19**, 182–7.

Johnstone, I. B. and Crane, S. (1986). Haemostatic abnormalities in horse with colic – their prognostic value. *Equine Vet. J.*, **18**, 271–4.

MacDonald, M. H., Pascoe, J. R., Stover, S. M. and Meagher, D. M. (1989). Survival after small intestinal resection and anastomosis in horses. *Vet. Surg.*, **18**, 415–23.

McCarthy, R. N. and Hutchins, D. R. (1988). Survival rates and post-operative complications after equine colic surgery. *Aus.Vet. J.*, **65**, 40–43.

Moore, J. N., Owen, R. R. and Lumsden, J. H. (1976). Clinical evaluation of blood lactate levels in equine colic. *Equine Vet. J.*, **8**, 49–54.

Moore, R. M., Hance, S. R., Hardy, J. *et al.* (1994). Colonic luminal pressure in horses with strangulating or non-strangulating obstruction of the large colon. *Vet. Surg.*, **23**, 411.

Orsini, J. A., Elser, A. H., Galligan, D. T. and Donawick, W. J. (1988). Prognostic index for equine acute abdominal crisis (colic). *Am. J. Vet. Res.*, **49**, 1969–71.

Parker, J. E., Fubini, S. L. and Todhunter, R. J. (1989). Retrospective evaluation of repeat celiotomy in 53 horses with acute gastrointestinal disease. *Vet. Surg.*, **18**, 424–31.

Parry, B. W., Anderson, G. A. and Gay, C. C. (1983). Prognosis in equine colic: A study of individual variables used in case assessment. *Equine Vet. J.*, **15**, 337–44.

Parry, B. W., Anderson, G. A. and Gay, C. C. (1983). Prognosis in equine colic: a comparative study of variables used to assess individual colic cases. *Equine Vet. J.*, **15(3)**, 211–15.

Parry, B. W. (1986). Prognostic evaluation of equine colic cases. *Compend. Cont. Ed.*, **8**, 98–104.

Parry, B. W. (1987). Use of clinical pathology in evaluation of horses with colic. *Vet. Clin. N. Am. Equine Pract.*, **3**, 529–42.

Philips, T. J. and Walmsley, J. P. (1993). Retrospective analysis of the results of 151 exploratory laparotomies in horses with gastrointestinal disease. *Equine Vet. J.*, **25**, 427–31.

Puotenen-Reinert, A. (1986). Study of variables commonly used in examination of equine colic cases to assess prognostic value. *Equine Vet. J.*, **18**, 275–7.

Reeves, M. J., Hilbert, B. J. and Morris, R. S. (1986). A retrospective study of 320 colic cases referred to a veterinary teaching hospital. *Proc. Equine Colic Res. Symp.*, **2**, 242–50, Veterinary Learning Systems.

Reeves, M. J., Curtis, C. R., Salman, M. D. and Stashak, T. S. (1987). Descriptive epidemiology and risk factors indicating the need for surgery and evaluation of prognosis. Morris Animal Foundation Colic Study. *Proc. Am. Assoc. Equine Pract. Ann. Conv.*, pp. 83–96.

Reeves, M. J., Curtis, C. R., Salman, M. D. *et al.* (1990). A multivariable prognostic model for equine colic patients. *Prev. Vet. Med.*, **9**, 241–57.

White, N. A. and Lessard, P. (1986). Risk factors and clinical signs associated with cases of equine colic. *Proc. Am. Assoc. Equine Pract. Ann. Conv.*, pp. 637–44.

6 Husbandry and prevention

Diet and management

Horses on pasture are 'trickle feeders' and graze almost continuously for up to 17 hours per day, with breaks at distinct periods between 3.30 am and 4.30 am (Pond *et al.*, 1993). The very specialist large intestine of the horse has developed to allow it to thrive on a high-fibre diet. The stomach and small intestine, which have evolved to digest soluble nutrients, function to reduce time spent by fibre in these segments before delivering it rapidly to the large intestine (Pagan *et al.*, 1997). Domestication imposes highly artificial conditions on this delicate process, and could be responsible for many gastrointestinal diseases. Deviation from a grazing pattern can lead to gastric ulceration and, possibly through disturbances in the enterosystemic cycle, to colic (Freeman, 1997). Other factors that can play an important part in altering digestive tract function are the digestibility of grains, the nature of the pasture and access to water.

The magnitude of the digestive secretions in this species following a single large meal is sufficient to activate the renin–angiotension system (Argenzio, 1990). The resulting aldosterone secretion can increase water and ion absorption from the colon, which could dehydrate the colonic contents and cause impaction colic (Clarke *et al.*, 1990).

The enterosystemic cycle refers to the production of fluid necessary for digestion of nutrients by the intestine and the recovery of almost all that fluid by small and, to a greater extent, large intestinal absorptive processes (Argenzio, 1975; Clarke *et al.*, 1990). In order to maintain normal gastrointestinal water balance, total net absorption from the intestine is approximately 98 per cent of the combined intake and endogenous secretions, a volume equivalent to a horse's extracellular fluid space. Most water resorption takes place in the large intestine. Diarrhoea may result from failure to recover this fluid, while recovery of too much may lead to impaction colic (Argenzio, 1975; Clarke *et al.*, 1990). Episodic feeding of horses (i.e. twice a day) can result in a 15 per cent decrease in plasma volume at each feeding, compared with horses fed continuously, apparently caused by abrupt loss of fluid into the intestine during production of normal digestive tract secretions (Clarke *et al.*, 1990).

Digestion in the small intestine is dependent on pancreatic and biliary secretions as well as mucosal enzymes and transport mechanisms. In contrast, the large intestine possesses neither mucosal enzymes nor transport mechanisms for amino acids, hexoses or B vitamins. Therefore, digestion and absorption of carbohydrate and protein depend upon the action of a flourishing microbial population in the large intestine.

Availability of substrate, prolonged retention time, anaerobic conditions and the ability to maintain an optimum pH in the face of continued addition of acidic end products of bacterial fermentation provide the necessary physiologic conditions to sustain this type of digestion.

Regardless of the source of dietary carbohydrate, the end products of fermentation in the colon are primarily volatile fatty acids (acetate, propionate and butyrate) and the gases carbon dioxide (CO_2) and methane (CH_4).

Only small amounts of lactate are produced under normal conditions, because lactic acid formed from soluble carbohydrate is metabolized to VFA when the microbes become adapted to a high grain ration. In addition, the colonic buffer systems maintain a pH at a level that favours the production of VFA rather than lactate. Despite the rapid absorption of VFA, animals fed at 12-hourly intervals demonstrate periods of VFA production in the large colon that exceed the absorptive capacity, whereas this is not the case in horses fed continuously. During these periods of rapid VFA production the colonic mucosa must secrete fluid and buffer to maintain the luminal pH, a process that is a critical function in preserving homeostasis.

One of the most important functions of the equine large intestine is the storage and absorption of tremendous volumes of water. Short chain fatty acids appear to play a major role in this process. Large volumes of water rich in Na^+ and HCO_3^- are exchanged across the colonic mucosa in cyclic periods of net influx and efflux apparently resulting from a cyclic pattern of microbial digestion (Argenzio, 1975).

Feeds or feeding activity have long been blamed for colic, but much of the information about diet and colic is based on hypothesis or extrapolation from experimental data that have not been substantiated by epidemiological observations. Moreover, epidemiological studies have yielded conflicting results. A significant decrease in risk of colic has been reported in horses at pasture and allowed to graze continuously (Reeves *et al.*, 1996). The risk is further diminished if horses on lush spring grass with a high moisture, low fibre content are provided with hay (Pagan *et al.*, 1997; Reeves *et al.*, 1996). Types of grass and hay such as poor quality roughage or coastal Bermuda hay are suspected of causing colic in groups of horses, as is overfeeding of grain.

Epidemiological studies in Virginia–Maryland (Tinker *et al.*, 1997) and Texas (Cohen *et al.*, 1996) identified an increased risk of colic when feed type, grain or hay was changed. The Virginia–Maryland study documented an increased risk of colic in horses fed mixed grains such as sweat feed and pelleted grains compared with horses fed single grains or no grain. This study also reported that daily feeding of concentrate of 2.5–5 kg/day and more than 5 kg/day increased the risk of colic 4.3 and

6.3 times respectively compared with horses fed no grain. In contrast, Reeves *et al.* (1996) found that horses with colic were fed less concentrates than controls. The amount of grain rather than the type of grain is probably the most important factor, but the increased risk observed for horses fed any type of mixed grain requires further investigation.

Feeding small amounts of grain at frequent intervals has been reported to reduce the fluid shifts in the large colon seen with twice-daily feeding. Although no correlation was found between feeding frequency and colic in the North Carolina study, feeding more than twice daily increased the risk of colic in the Virginia–Maryland study. A greater daily increase of grain, rather than the frequency of feeding, was the likely explanation for this. The mechanism by which grain causes intestinal problems is not fully understood, but it is speculated to be the result of feeding high levels of soluble carbohydrate that can alter the microbial population, intraluminal hydration or pH of the caecum or colon. Grain concentrates contain large amounts of starch, which is digested by enzymes in the small intestine to form simple sugars for absorption by the small intestinal mucosa. Digestibility varies, however, with 84 per cent of starch derived from oats being digested in the small intestine compared with 29 per cent from corn (Meyer *et al.*, 1993). Any starch that escapes digestion in the small intestine is converted to lactic acid by microbial fermentation in the large intestine. This can lower pH to levels that can damage the mucosa and change bacterial flora (Argenzio, 1975), leading to colic or laminitis. To avoid these complications, grain should be processed by steam crimping, rolling and grinding to improve small intestinal digestibility (Pagan *et al.*, 1997). No more than 2–3 kg should be fed in a single meal, and grain meals should be spread throughout the day. Dietary fat can be used as an alternative energy source to some grain, and oats is preferable to other grains (Pagan *et al.*, 1997).

Changes in diet, both grain and hay, are related to increased risk of colic. Cohen *et al.* (1996) reported that a recent (within 2 weeks) change in diet was associated with doubling the risk of colic, irrespective of changes in stabling or exercise. Tinker *et al.* (1997) reported that the incidence of colic was higher on farms where horses had six or more diet changes per year. Due to the fact that diet is widely regarded as an important risk factor for colic, dietary practices can be modified to decrease risk. It is apparent from the little reliable information available that epidemiologic studies of diet and colic are much needed.

Horses that have access to pasture or drylot without constant access to water have a significantly increased risk of colic (Reeves *et al.*, 1996). Horse owners and stable managers should be appraised of this need for a constant supply of fresh water. Due to the fact that horses are continuous feeders and consume a high-fibre diet, both small and large intestinal digestive processes demand enormous volumes of digestive secretions (Clarke *et al.*, 1990). Failure to replace this fluid by providing a constant supply of water can lead to increased absorption of water by the colon, thus dehydrating colonic contents, with risk of impaction.

Management practices have been associated with an increased risk of colic. Reports have suggested that sudden decreases in activity such as curtailing regular exercise or changing from turnout activity to strict stall confinement because of injury or after surgery increased the risk of caecal or colon impaction. The study carried out by Reeves *et al.* (1996) demonstrated that horses at pasture were significantly more likely to have colic than stall-confined horses, although the risk of colic in pastured animals decreased if horses had access to two or three pastures. Proudman (1991), in a study carried out in the United Kingdom, found that recent changes in management, the most common being providing access to lush pasture, was the most frequently reported putative risk factor for spasmodic/undiagnosed colic. Tinker *et al.* (1994) observed that horses used for racing or eventing, or those in active training, were at increased risk of colic relative to horses used for other activities, but these activities did not pose an increased risk when compared to other factors. Other studies and individual observations have suggested that, when horses change from an active exercise schedule to minimal activity due to stall confinement (often for medical reasons), they are predisposed to impaction colic (Dabareiner and White, 1995).

Parasites

Strongylus vulgaris

Perhaps the best known parasite-associated colic is that of the early migratory stages of the large strongyle *Strongylus vulgaris*, which was once claimed to cause 90 per cent of all colic cases. Since the introduction of effective larvicidal anthelmintics, however, the prevalence of this parasite is much reduced, and is seen in fewer than 4 per cent of all horses undergoing autopsy (Love, 1997). Large strongyles are regarded as the most pathogenic of the equine internal parasites, with *S. vulgaris* being regarded as the most injurious. The life cycle is similar to that of the small strongyles. Adults attach to the caecum and ventral colon. Ingested *S. vulgaris* larvae migrate from the gut through the submucosal arterioles to the caecal and colic arteries, reaching the cranial mesenteric artery within 4 months. They then return to the intestine via the lumina of the arteries. The prepatent period is 6–7 months. *S. vulgaris* exerts its injurious effects by causing extensive damage to the endothelium of the blood vessels along its course of migration and inducing thrombosis. Non-strangulating infarction can result from reduced blood flow to a segment of intestine, which is caused by an intravascular occlusion, almost always a thrombus or an embolus. The occlusion occurs primarily in the cranial mesenteric artery and/or its branches; the ileocaecocolic branch is the most commonly occluded. Partial occlusion of these arteries leads to diminished intestinal blood flow and reduced tissue perfusion, especially in the ileum, caecum and large colon. In general, the effects are impaired digestion and absorption and reduced motility. These changes cause varying degrees of abdominal discomfort, depending on the extent of the hypoperfused tissue. It has frequently been suggested that the hypoxia resulting from this vascular damage may lead to more serious colic through the development of intussusception, volvulus or mesenteric hernias, but this has never been proved. The most commonly recognized sequel to verminous thrombosis is focal or multifocal infarction of the ileum, caecum or colon. The classic concept that this is the result of emboli breaking away from the central thrombus and lodging in peripheral branches of the ileocaecocolic artery must be questioned on the basis of both experimental and clinical information. Following experimental infection in foals, infarction occurred as the result of thrombosis of small arterioles and not of embolization from the cranial mesenteric artery (Georgi, 1973). Similar studies on 18 naturally occurring cases of intestinal infarction associated with thrombosis of the mesenteric vasculature did not support gross peripheral embolization of thrombi as the predominant cause (White, 1981).

Thromboxane produced by platelets aggregating in the damaged arteries induces vasoconstriction and focal ischaemia, and may explain the frequent infarctions in which no evidence of an embolus can be found in the arteries that supply the infarcted area (White, 1981). This reaction may also be responsible for some of the mild colic cases attributed to *S. vulgaris*.

Most thrombi or emboli are small and cause only transient ischaemia as collateral circulation re-establishes circulation to the affected segment of bowel. If the ischaemic lesion is so extensive, however, that it cannot be spanned by collateral circulation, it becomes infarcted and necrotic, triggering the same morphologic and biochemical changes as described for strangulation obstruction. Horses with non-strangulating infarction show signs of slowly progressing colic dullness and depression. Gastric reflux due to ileus occurs in 50 per cent of horses with caecal or colon infarction. Peritoneal fluid shows a significant increase in proteins and a progressive increase in neutrophils as necrosis of the infarcted area progresses and endotoxins and bacteria leak into the peritoneal cavity. Vascular collapse and death usually occur within 24–48 hours of the onset of clinical signs.

Mild cases may respond to antibiotic therapy, but when deterioration in clinical parameters indicate more extensive infarction, surgery offers the only means of saving the horse's life. Focal lesions at the pelvic flexure or at other locations in the left colon can be resected, as can infarction of the caecum when limited to the apex. Infarction may, however, subsequently develop at locations that were apparently normal at laparotomy. Cases in which infarction involves the base of the caecum, the origin of the right ventral colon or the distal right dorsal colon are inoperable.

Control

Due to the long prepatent period of 26 weeks, larval development is completed during the winter months (Duncan, 1974; Ogbourne, 1971). Therefore, horses should receive larvicidal treatment (5 day's fenbendazole or ivermectin) during the autumn and winter in addition to regular worming in the grazing season. This will prevent *S. vulgaris* egg output rising in the spring and thereafter.

Cyathostomes

Recent quantitative epidemiological studies have confirmed that cyathostome infections can be associated with the occurrence of mild, medical forms of equine colic. Uhlinger (1990), in a 3-year prospective study, showed that the incidence of colic on farms on which cyathostomes were not successfully controlled was much greater than on those on which parasite prophylaxis was effective. Over 50 species of small strongyles that affect horses exist. The life cycle is direct, with females laying eggs that are passed in the faeces, where they develop into infective larvae and are ingested by grazing horses. Once in the intestine, infective larvae invade the wall of the caecum and large colon, develop into the next larval stage and remain in the gut wall for 1–2 months. Larvae then emerge into the gut lumen and mature into adults. The pathogenic mechanisms by which parasites cause colic are not known, but in experimental studies it has been shown that both large and small strongyle larvae can give rise to alterations in intestinal motility. This change in motility may reflect either a direct physical effect of the larvae or, perhaps more likely, an indirect effect via release of immunochemical mediators that affect either intestinal smooth muscle and/or intestinal vasculature. A recent case report implicated cyathostomes rather than large strongyles infection with non-strangulating infarction (Mair, 1994).

Cyathostome infections are a cause of protein-losing enteropathy, with a typical presentation of rapid, marked weight loss, most usually in young animals in late winter or early spring. This condition is often referred to as acute larval cyathostomosis. The condition does, however, occur in horses of all ages and at all times of the year, and there is a trend towards increased occurrence during late autumn (Love, 1997). Cyathostomosis constitutes typhlitis and colitis as the result of the host reaction to large numbers of larvae either entering or synchronously emerging from the intestinal mucosa. It may occur as a sporadic, individual animal condition or, less frequently, it may affect several animals on the same premises. In addition to rapid weight loss, many affected animals develop additional signs such as peripheral oedema and/or fever and marked lethargy. Some cases develop sudden onset of diarrhoea. A mild form of cyathostomosis with vague malaise, fever and anorexia is recognized fairly commonly in the UK, but it is difficult to establish the true prevalence due to difficulties in positively diagnosing this form of the condition (Love, 1997). Clinical cyathostomosis commonly occurs in animals that are subjected to a parasite prophylaxis programme. In the UK, cyathostomosis is the most common cause of diarrhoea in young and adult horses (but not foals). Recent anthelmintic dosing is a predisposing factor for this type of diarrhoea. It has been hypothesized that a negative feedback mechanism exists between luminal cyathostomes and larvae within the mucosa, which contributes to their arrested development. Anthelmintic treatment results in death and expulsion of the luminal worms, but the mucosal larvae are spared and, free from the negative feedback mechanism, synchronously resume development, resulting in typhlitis and colitis. This effect may also apply to cyathostome-associated weight loss. When one member of a grazing

Table 6.1 Treatment of clinical cyathostomosis

	Dose rate	*Day*
Fenbendazole	7.5 mg/kg bw sid	1–5
		16–20
		31–35
Ivermectin	0.2 mg/kg bw	6
		21
		36
Prednisolone	1 mg/kg bw sid (am)	20–40
	1 mg/kg bw eod (am)	20–40

group of horses has overt clinical cyathostomosis, the others are likely to carry a large cyathostome burden. Under these circumstances it would appear logical to treat the entire group, but it should be recognized that this carries the potential of inducing further clinical cases.

Treatment of clinical cyathostomosis is based on intensive anthelmintic medication and concurrent corticosteroid therapy (Table 6.1).

Moxidectin at 0.4 mg/kg bw at 10-day intervals may be an alternative therapy to the anthelmintics in Table 6.1, but as yet there is no published data to support its use in clinical cases (Abbot, 1998).

The same treatment regimen is used for horses with cyathostome-associated diarrhoea, with additional medication with codeine phosphate elixir at a dose rate of approximately 3 mg/kg bw tid (days 1–9), 2 mg/kg bw tid (days 10–14) and 1 mg/kg bw tid (days 15–20) (Love, 1997).

The equine tapeworm (*Anoplocephala perfoliata*)

Until recently, the equine tapeworm *Anoplocephala perfoliata* was difficult to diagnose and was considered to be of questionable pathogenicity by pathologists, who regarded its presence in the intestinal tract of the horses at *postmortem* as incidental.

Infection in the live horse usually went undetected because of difficulties associated with coprological diagnosis, and because no clearly defined clinical symptoms were associated with it. In the 1980s, a number of case reports cited circumstantial evidence suggesting that this tapeworm was associated with the development of certain 'intestinal accidents' in the horse, which included intussusceptions, ileal hypertrophy, caecal hypertrophy at the ileocaecal orifice, ileal and caecal perforation (Table 6.2). Recent studies have defined the pathology caused by this parasite, and novel approaches to *antemortem* diagnosis have provided a tool for epidemiological studies.

Anoplocephala perfoliata is a cestode with an indirect life cycle via pasture dwelling oribatid mites. The parasite matures to an adult in 6–10 weeks, and attains a final size of only 5–8 cm in length. It has a pre-

Table 6.2 Accidents associated with *Anoplocephala perfoliata*

Ileal hypertrophy and perforation	Edwards, 1986
Intussusceptions	Barclay *et al.*, 1982; Beroza *et al.*, 1986; Cosgrove *et al.*, 1986; Edwards, 1986; Owen *et al.*, 1989; Gaugan, 1990
Caecal perforation	Beroza *et al.*, 1983, 1980
Caecal torsion	Beroza *et al.*, 1986

dilection for the ileocaecal region, where it attaches to the mucosa by means of suckers on the scolex, obtaining its nutrition by absorption through its cuticle. In a study reported by Fogarty *et al.* (1994), 51 per cent of tapeworms were attached to the mucosa at the ileocaecal junction and/or caecum; 5 per cent only at the ileocaecal junction, 24 per cent only to the caecal mucosa, and 22 per cent at both sites.

Pathological studies have identified both gross and histological pathology at the site of parasite attachment on and around the ileocaecal junction, the severity of pathology being directly proportional to the number of parasites present. The greatest damage is seen when large numbers of tapeworms are clustered together. Pearson *et al.* (1993) showed that, when more than 100 tapeworms were present, there was ulceration of the mucosa (sometimes extending into the submucosa), local mucosal haemorrhage/diphtheresis, and infiltration of the mucosa, lamina propria and submucosa with eosinophils and lymphocytes. These inflammatory responses extended beyond the area of the lesion. The mechanism by which this pathology arises remains uncertain, but it is reasonable to implicate parasite-derived antigens in the process.

Adult parasites shed gravid proglottids, which break up during passage through the large intestine. The eggs are very characteristic in appearance but, unfortunately, are present in very small numbers in the faeces of infected horses. Validation studies report sensitivities of 11–61 per cent, indicating that the conventional centrifugal/flotation technique is an inadequate method for diagnosing equine cestodiasis. The need for an improved diagnostic method has led to the development of a successful IgG(T) ELISA, using excretory/secretory antigens, for the serodiagnosis of tapeworms in horses (Proudman and Trees, 1996). Although it showed only a slight improvement in overall sensitivity, it shows a good correlation between ELISA optical density values and infection intensity in individual animals. This is of considerable importance, because intestinal helminth disease is not related to the presence or absence of parasites (prevalence) but to the infection intensity (number of tapeworms).

Clinically based evidence is insufficient to unequivocally implicate *Anoplocephala perfoliata* in ileocaecal colic. A case–control study (Proudman and Edwards, 1993) using coprologic-diagnosis reported an association, but the information was limited by low diagnostic sensitivity.

The IgG(T) ELISA has offered a unique opportunity to conduct other case–control studies.

In a case–control study in the UK, there was evidence that colic cases had a significantly greater titre to *A. perfoliata* than age-matched controls from the same premises which did not experience colic. In the same study, it was estimated that 81 per cent of ileal impactions and 22 per cent of mild medical 'spasmodic colics' were tapeworm-associated (Proudman *et al.*, 1998).

Although prevalence is usually high, most infected horses have low burdens and are therefore at low risk. Elimination of tapeworms is probably not possible and is unnecessary. Control methods should be aimed at identifying and treating the minority of horses with high infection intensities.

Most commercially-available anthelmintics have no activity against *A. perfoliata*. Praziquantel and niclosamide have proven anticestode activity, but niclosamide was found to have poor efficacy at a dose rate of 50 mg/kg bwt (Slocombe, 1979). Neither of these drugs is available in a form licensed for use in the horse. The only licensed equine anthelmintic with known efficacy against *A. perfoliata* is pyrantel. Pyrantel salts have an efficacy against tapeworms of 13–100 per cent, depending upon the experimental method employed, when administered at twice the anti-nematode dose (i.e. 38 mg/kg bwt) for pyrantel emboate. An average efficacy for pyrantel pamoate of 93 per cent against tapeworms has been reported (Lyons *et al.*, 1986). Critical trials suggest that pyrantel causes complete removal of tapeworms from the intestinal tract, and not just removal of mature segments leaving the scolex attached. A novel anthelmintic regimen that has been used in North America is continuous low-level dosing with pyrantel salts as feed additives (Reinemeyer, 1998). Whether such a regimen is successful against tapeworms has yet to be evaluated.

The role of tapeworms in equine colic should be kept in perspective. They represent a small but avoidable risk factor in the aetiology of certain types of colic, so all horse owners should be encouraged to incorporate appropriate anthelmintics in their deworming programmes. Recent studies (Fogarty *et al.*, 1994) suggest there is little variation in the prevalence of infection or number of parasites present throughout the year because the oribatid mite survives both on the pasture and in forage and bedding during the winter months.

Parascaris equorum

Heavy infestations of *Parascaris equorum* in foals, weanlings and yearlings can lead to small intestinal impaction, particularly after the administration of a high efficacy anthelmintic such as ivermectin, piperazine or an organophosphate. Ascarid impaction can lead to colic, toxaemia, intestinal perforation or rupture, peritonitis, abscessation and intussusception of the small intestine.

Although *P. equorum* infection is common, with a prevalence of 31–61 per cent (Haas, 1979) in horses younger than 1 year, ascarid impactions are an uncommon cause of colic. Unlike other species, intra-uterine infection does not occur, and most foals are infected soon after birth, regardless of management factors. Sucklings, weanlings and yearlings are most likely to develop ascarid impactions. A prevalence of 25 per cent has been reported in animals over 1 year of age. Horses older than 6 months develop an immunity, even if they have not been exposed to ascarids (Clayton and Duncan, 1978).

In a retrospective study, the median age for foals with ascarid impactions was 5 months (range to 24 months), and most of these foals were impacted with adult worms. However, the larvae, which are only a few millimetres long when they return to the small intestine, will grow into mature worms 10–50 cm long and 3–5 mm in diameter in 6–12 weeks. They grow much more rapidly than the foal's intestine, so that animals with heavy infections frequently have impactions with immature worms.

In a recent retrospective study by Southwood *et al.* (1996), 75 per cent of the impactions in foals occurred in the autumn, and recent worming was not a consistent finding.

Diagnosis

A definitive diagnosis is made either at surgery or autopsy, but a tentative diagnosis of ascarid impaction may be made on the basis of clinical signs in young horses with a poor worming history and the presence of larval or mature ascarid worms in faeces or gastric reflux. Impactions may exist, however, in animals with negative faecal and gastric reflux findings. Other non-specific findings included distended small intestine on rectal examination and abnormal peritoneal fluid, but eosinophilia is not found in foals with ascarid impaction. The result of faecal egg counts must be interpreted with care. Although the presence of eggs proves the animal has an ascarid infection, egg counts do not accurately reflect worm burden because of the extreme fecundity of the mature ascarids and because immature worms, which can cause impaction, do not produce eggs. The maturity of the worms, anthelmintic treatment, host immunity and competition between ascarids for available nutrients all influence egg production (Clayton and Duncan, 1978).

Treatment

Horses with mild colic attributed to ascarids may be treated medically with mineral oil, intravenous fluid therapy, anti-inflammatory drugs and analgesics, but, unless obstruction occurs, a definitive diagnosis is never reached.

The decision for surgery is usually based on persistent abdominal pain that does not respond to analgesics, nasogastric reflux abdominal distension and abnormal peritoneal fluid. In foals too small to allow rectal palpation, radiographs may demonstrate distended small intestine and round, opaque, intraluminal soft-tissue densities (Adair, 1990). Exploration of the abdomen via a midline laparotomy incision allows a positive diagnosis of impaction to be made. Although large numbers of ascarids may be found throughout the intestinal tract, impaction most commonly occurs in the distal small intestine, attributed to passage of dead or dying ascarids from the jejunum after anthelmintic treatment.

More than one enterotomy incision on the antimesenteric border of the small intestine may be necessary to relieve the impaction. The intestine is examined closely for evidence of vascular compromise, and any non-viable segment should be resected. Intestinal rupture or abscess can occur and necessitate euthanasia.

Post-operative survival

Survival of horses after surgery is poor. In one study (Southwood *et al.*, 1996), only five of ten foals with ascarid impaction survived long enough to be discharged from the hospital, and only one of ten survived long-term (at least 2 years). Two retrospective studies reported overall survival rates of 45 per cent (Cable *et al.*, 1996) and 43 per cent (Vasitas *et al.*, 1996). Post-operative complications are common, and include recurrent colic, endotoxaemia, adhesions, diffuse peritonitis, focal necrotizing enteritis and intestinal perforation. The reason for this poor prognosis is not known. Ascarids in the intestine may cause damage to the intestinal wall, which may not appear significant at surgery. Intestinal ischaemia may result from distension, or possibly from the effects of toxins from the ascarids (Southwood *et al.*, 1996). Absorption of highly antigenic fluid released into the intestine when the cuticle of *P. equorum* ruptures following organophosphate anthelmintics reportedly causes ileus and secondary impaction (Uhlinger and Brumbaugh, 1990). Chronic debilitation associated with severe ascarid burdens may be another factor in the poor survival rate. Not all the ascarids present in the intestinal tract are removed at surgery, and those remaining may cause further intestinal damage and release toxins. Whether or not anthelmintic treatment should be administered after surgery is controversial. If it is, it should be preceded by mineral oil to promote the passage of the dead ascarids and decrease the absorption of ascarid derived toxins (Southwood *et al.*, 1996).

Prevention

The fecundity of the parasite (a mature female can produce 200 000 eggs per day) and the persistence of the eggs in the environment due to their sticky outer coat and thick wall make complete prevention of ascarid infection unfeasible. However, reducing the degree of exposure by reducing egg numbers is important (Clayton, 1986). Preventative regimens involve regular deworming and monitoring of the mare and foal, and minimizing ascarid eggs in the environment (Austin *et al.*, 1990; Clayton, 1986; Di Pietro and Todd, 1988). Foals should be dewormed at 6 weeks of age, at which time they should be included in the deworming programme used on the farm.

Most broad spectrum anthelmintics such as invermectin and fenbendazole are 90–100 per cent effective against ascarids. Thiabendazole is relatively ineffective against ascarids. Although no anthelmintic is effective against ascarids during their migration, many are effective against all the intestinal stages, making it possible to kill the worms while they are still small. Ascarid infections are treated by medication with either ivermectin (0.2 mg/kg) or fenbendazole (10 mg/kg for 5 consecutive days).

Parasite prophylaxis

Equine parasite control programmes are intended to reduce parasite transmission by minimizing contact between horses and the infective stages of parasites in their environment. Consequently, horses on control programmes are less likely to suffer damage or clinical disease due to parasitic infestations. Appropriate selection and utilization of effective anthelmintic, good management practices to reduce parasite transmission and assessment of parasite control are essential components of a complete parasite control programme (Di Pietro, 1992).

The nematode species of primary importance have changed during the past decade in developed regions of the world because of the advent of highly efficient anthelmintics. As indicated earlier, their use has reduced the prevalence of *Strongylus vulgaris*, the most pathogenic of internal parasites. With the effective control of large strongyles, more attention has focused on the cyathostomes. Deworming programmes for adult horses are primarily aimed at controlling large and small strongyles and bots. Programmes for horses less than 1 year old are directed at the control of *P. equorum*, large and small strongyles and bots. Tapeworm and *Strongyloides westeri* control is necessary on premises with a past history of infestations.

No single parasite control strategy is ideal for all horses under all management conditions, or for use in all regional environments. Therefore, a number of different but inter-related factors must be taken into consideration before deciding on a programme that suits individual needs.

The focus of most control strategies is the regular use of anthelmintics, but the overuse of these drugs has raised concern recently because of the potential for the induction of drug-resistant strains of cyathostomes.

Anthelmintics

Six major classes of anthelmintics are currently available for use in the horse (Table 6.3), the most useful and widely used of these being the avermectins, benzimidazoles and pyrimidines. Many of the others listed are less useful because they have a reduced spectrum of activity and lower safety indices.

Avermectins

The avermectins are macrocyclic lactones that disrupt the neuromuscular function of nematodes and arthropods. Ivermectin, the avermectin currently available for use in the horse, has a wide range of activities at a low dose. Its activity against adult and migrating nematode larvae and all stages of Gasterophilus species larvae is unique. It is not effective against Anoplocephala tapeworm species or the encysted larvae of the cyathostomes. Cyathostome eggs normally reappear in faeces 8–10 weeks after treatment with ivermectin, but this period may be shorter in younger stock, which are likely to be more heavily infected. Moxidectin, which has a range of activity similar to ivermectin and activity against encysted cyathostome larvae, has been introduced for use in horses in the United States and Europe.

Table 6.3 Six major classes of anthelmintics currently available for use in the horse

| Drug class | Anthelmintic | Relative onset of action | Dosage (mg/kg) | Method | Mean efficiency | | Parascaris equorum | Anoplocephala perfoliata | Bots |
					Large Strongyles	Small Strongyles			
Avermectin	Ivermectin	Slow	0.2	S.O.	100	100	100	None	99
Avermectin	Moxidectin Not in foals < 4 months. Not in debilitated horses	Slow	0.4	O	100	100	100	None	90
Benzimidazole	Thiabendazole	Slow	44–48	S.F.O.	97	95	42	None	None
	Mebendazole	Slow	8.8	S.F.O.	80–97	87	08	None	None
	Fenbendazole	Slow	7.5 routine worming 30.0 for cyathostome 7.5 for 5 days for migrating strongyle larvae	S.F.O.	95–97	97	85	Limited	None
	Oxibendazole	Slow	10–15	S.O.	97	97	85	?	None
Pyrimidine	Pyrantel pamoate Pyrantel tartrate	Slow Slow	19 38 (for tapeworms)	S.F.O.	70–77	95	95	90	None
Imidazothiazole	Levamisole-piperazine	Fast	8/88	S	63–97	97	100	None	None
Organophosphate	Trichlorfon	Fast	40	8.0	0	0	97	None	95

S, stomach tube; F, feed; O, oral paste or drench

Benzimidazoles

A number of benzimidazoles are available in various formulations and mixtures for use in the horse. These compounds are highly effective against most nematodes living within the gastrointestinal tract, although there is some variation in the spectrum of activity. Some benzimidazoles have been demonstrated to be highly effective against migrating large strongyles and encysted cyathostome larvae when used at increased dose rates for prolonged periods, e.g. fenbendazole at 10 mg/kg for 5 days. Cyathostome resistance to benzimidazoles has been documented.

Pyrimidines

The pyrimidines licensed for use in the horse are pyrantel pamoate and pyrantel tartrate. The pyrantel salts are unique in that they are effective against the common tapeworm *Anoplocephala perfoliata*. Its efficacy is raised to more than 90 per cent when used at twice the recommended dosage for nematode control.

Pyrantel tartrate, the most recently introduced pyrimidine, is used as a daily food supplement and functions in a prophylactic manner. In most circumstances, this method of delivery has proved very effective. However, its effectiveness in foals that are heavily challenged may be reduced, and its use in young animals also eliminates or delays the development of acquired immunity in the animals. Prophylaxis against tapeworm with daily administration of pyrantel tartrate has not been confirmed.

Parasite control

Several alternative parasite prophylaxis programmes have been shown to be effective, if carefully and precisely managed, but there is inherent potential for complications if strategic or daily in-fed programmes are utilized without strict supervision (Love, 1997).

Level of control

The degree of parasite control necessary to maintain optimal health in a given horse is dependent on its age, its use, management conditions, stocking rates and its potential exposure to horses with heavy infections. Although two anthelmintic treatments per year might be adequate to maintain adult horses used for recreation and maintained at low stocking rates of less than one horse per acre in excellent health, such a programme is not suitable for athletic horses or mares on a large breeding farm (Klei, 1997). Variations can occur even within such environments.

Climate

Seasonal climatic variations in temperature and rainfall affect the development and survival of larvae on pasture and, thus, pasture infectivity. In northern temperate regions, where severe winters reduce pasture infectivity, the major period of strongyle transmission is during the summer months. In these regions, strongyle infections in mature horses can be controlled by strategic therapy to remove luminal parasites during the spring and early summer, which reduces pasture contamination and re-infection. In contrast, in tropical and semi-tropical regions, high temperatures during the summer months reduce the survival of larvae on pasture, and the optimal period of transmission is during the cooler winter months. In these environments it may be possible to eliminate summer treatments in adult horses.

Drug resistance

It is unlikely that there will be any new group of anthelmintics for horses in the next 10–15 years, so it is important that the efficacy of the existing ones is preserved for as long as possible. Resistance to anthelmintics in the horse is limited to the cyathostomes. On a worldwide basis, there is widespread resistance to benzimidazoles and some resistance to pyrantel. Although benzimidazole-resistant cyathostomes were shown for a time to be susceptible to oxibendazole, prolonged, widespread use has, not surprisingly, caused resistance to this drug to develop as well. Resistance has a genetic basis, and frequent, repeated use of the same class of anthelmintic selects for resistant populations. There have been no definite reports of resistance to ivermectin in horses despite its repeated and sometimes excessive use in some farms, and the fact that resistance against trichostrongyle nematodes has been demonstrated in ruminants. A possible explanation for the lack of ivermectin resistance may be related to the large number of cyathostomes that escape ivermectin selection pressure, including those hypobiotic and developing larvae encysted in the mucosa, which may be more than 80 per cent of the total worm burden (Klei, 1997).

The efficiency of anthelmintic treatment should be checked by carrying out a faecal egg count reduction (ECR) test on a representative number of horses, all of which must have egg counts of less than 200 eggs/g before treatment commenced. The egg counts should be carried out on the day of worming and 7 days after treatment with pyrantel, 10–14 days following benzimidazoles and 21 days after ivermectin, to allow for the egg reappearance periods of the drugs. Products that fail to reduce egg counts by 90 per cent are indicating a degree of resistance. If the ECR test clearly identifies resistance, the anthelmintic in question should be removed from the April to September grazing programme, but should be retained for strategic dosing, where its action is unique.

Control programmes

Interval or suppressive treatment

The majority of horse owners practise parasite control by use of interval treatment during the period of the year that the animals are at pasture – in temperate climates, this is essentially the whole year. The underlying principle of interval dosing is to suppress output of eggs in faeces, and hence prevent contamination of pasture with infective stages of parasites. Reasons for failure of interval dosing programmes include incorrect dosing intervals, lack of synchronization of dosing, anthelmintic resistance and acquisition of horses harbouring worm stages unaffected by standard anthelmintic dosing.

The dosing intervals in parasite prophylaxis programmes are established on the basis of the period for which faeces remain free of eggs

Table 6.4 Faecal egg count reduction test

Anthelmintic	Timing after treatment (days)
Pyrantel	7
Febendazole	10–14
Ivermectin	21

after dosing. This varies, however, with each anthelmintic class (Table 6.4), a fact which owners frequently do not appreciate. They consequently dose every 8 weeks, regardless of the product they are using. Prophylaxis programmes may appear to fail if animals are purchased with pre-existing burdens of mucosal cyathostomes and/or migrating stages of ascarids, which are much less susceptible to anthelmintics administered at standard rates employed in prophylactic programmes. Consequently, they may survive dosing and mature to give rise to disease at a later stage. If interval deworming is used, faecal egg counts on all horses is recommended to assess the effectiveness of the interval or to assess resistance to the anthelmintic.

Fast rotation

In fast rotation programmes, different classes of anthelmintics are alternated during the year at predetermined periods. They have the advantage of allowing for annual elimination of parasites, such as gasterophilus and Anoplocephala, which are not uniformly killed by all drugs. The rationale behind these programmes is that the increased interval between treatment with the same class of drug slows the development of resistance. Such rotational methods, however, have resulted in resistance to trichostrongyles in sheep under experimental conditions, and it is hypothesized that similar results could occur in horses.

Annual rotation

Annual rotation or slow rotation programmes employ the same anthelmintic at appropriate intervals throughout the year, based on ERP. Drug classes are alternated yearly. This approach may not be appropriate in all circumstances, because these programmes focus only on cyathostomes and do not take into account the variable efficacies of drugs against a broad range of parasites (Klei, 1997). The advantage of such programmes is that, theoretically, they minimize the potential risk of multiple drug-resistant cyathostome populations developing.

No rotation

This type of control involves the regular use of one effective drug until it no longer reduces cyathostome numbers as shown by faecal egg counts, and is generally restricted to the use of ivermectin or the low-dose feed additive formulation of pyrantel tartarate. It is easily implemented and provides for maximal reduction of parasite burdens. The rapid induction of drug resistance, which had been suggested might result from this type of programme, has not occurred with ivermectin. A significant delay in the development of acquired resistance is likely to accompany such management practices.

Seasonal or strategic programmes

A newer approach to the control of strongyles is the seasonal control programme, in which effective anthelmintics are used strategically to eliminate luminal cyathosomes before the season of the year that is optimal for the development of parasites on pasture. Pasture contamination, and thus re-infection, are reduced. Used in the spring and early summer at the appropriate interval for the anthelmintic used, and again in the autumn, these programmes have been effective in controlling cyathostomes in yearlings and mature horses in northern temperate regions. Similar programmes have been reported to be effective in the south-eastern regions of the United States by commencing these treatments in the early autumn (September) and discontinuing them in early spring (February/March). During the remainder of the year, climatic conditions limit any residual infective larva.

Daily anthelmintic in-feed programmes

Daily administration of 2.65 mg/kg of pyrantel tartrate is effective in the prevention of *S. vulgaris* infections and the control of large strongyles, small strongyles (adults and fourth-stage larvae in the intestine) and ascarids (adults and fourth-stage larvae in the intestine). Treatment on a daily basis with pyrantel tartrate kills larvae prior to their migration, and adult worms and larvae in the intestine. Since exclusive use of the same chemical class of compounds and frequent treatment virtually ensure the development of resistance, it could be argued that it is irresponsible to suppress parasitism too intensely. From a clinician's perspective, however, suppression offers maximal prevention (Reinemeyer, 1998).

Pasture management

Pasture management is critical, particularly with respect to faeces removal. The key elements of a successful programme are as follows:

1. Operate an overall system for the premises. The horse is often treated as an individual, even when grazing with what is effectively a herd of horses. Studies conducted among owners keeping horses on do-it-yourself livery premises show that only a third adopt any cohesive worming programme.
2. Utilize knowledge of the parasites' life cycles to enable strategic use to be made of the pasture available. Rotation of stock to clean pastures, particularly at times of the year when larval survival is expected to be minimal, may be an effective adjunct to anthelmintic control. Pasture space, however, is often limited, and moving horses to clean pasture following treatment may enhance the selection of drug-resistant populations of cyathostomes.

3. Treat young stock (foals, weanlings and yearlings) as a separate group. While regular worming with effective anthelmintics will usually keep output low in adult horses, this is not always the case for young stock. Without separate monitoring and excellent pasture management, the shorter egg reappearance time will lead to the build-up of damaging infection in young stock and on the pasture they graze.

Practical measures

1. Faeces removal is critical, particularly where there is young stock and/or heavy stocking densities. Twice-weekly mechanical removal of faeces in summer and once-weekly in November–March has been shown to have a beneficial effect in temperate regions (Herd, 1987), but it is labour intensive, and vacuum equipment for this purpose is expensive. The storage and disposal of large volumes of faeces in the absence of farm land to spread it on also poses a significant problem.
2. Harrowing pastures when the weather is dry is beneficial because it exposes infective larvae to desiccation and dramatically reduces larval survival time. Harrowing when wet, however, simply smears infective larvae all over the pasture, and should be avoided. Foals grazing harrowed pastures have been reported to have more parasites than those on pastures that were not harrowed (Slocombe, 1997).
3. With regard to stocking density, although a minimum of 1 acre per horse is desirable, it is common practice (particularly in the winter months) to have many more than one horse to the acre. Furthermore, most owners have only limited grazing at their disposal.
4. Cattle or sheep, either grazed with horses or moved in afterwards, will act as 'biohoovers', reducing the number of larvae on the pasture. They will also improve pasture quality by levelling grazing areas rejected by horses.
5. Strategic management of pasture should be employed, particularly for young stock, to reduce the risk posed by cyathostomes. In practice, this involves leaving pasture ungrazed by horses for at least 5 months from February onwards. By June any over-wintered larvae will have died off, therefore hay and silage aftermaths are ideal grazing.

Colic risk factors

Despite the practical and methodological challenges associated with conducting epidemiological studies of equine colic, the benefits of undertaking them are becoming increasingly evident. The results of these studies illustrate that risk factors for the disease do in fact exist and that colic, like most non-communicable diseases, is complex and multifactorial in nature.

A risk factor is an event, agent or phenomenon that is associated with a disease risk. Risk factors may be causal factors, predisposing factors, or simply indicators of a predisposing factor.

Some risk factors for colic that have been derived from clinical experience, descriptive case reports or hospitalized case series are included in Table 6.5. Most of these are markers of specific disease, and are accepted as risk factors even though conventional epidemiological

Table 6.5 Risk factors commonly associated with colic in horses

Factor	Disorder	Associated with:
Age	Meconium impaction	Young age (1–5 days)
	Ascaria impaction	Foals after recent worming
	Strangulating lipoma	Horses 23 years of age or older
	Epiploic foramen incarceration	Older horses
	Large colon torsion	Older age, mare's pregnancy
	Caecal impaction	Older horses
Breed	Inguinal hernia	Standard bred, warmblood and saddlebred stallions
	Large colon displacements	Large warmblood breeds
	Small colon obstruction	Ponies
Geographical location	Enteroliths	Highest incidence in California and Florida
	Ileal impaction	South-eastern United States
	Grass sickness	UK and Europe

analysis has not been completed to provide risk ratios and other direct evidence of causal relationship. More recently, the results of several epidemiological studies have been published. These include case–control studies by Reeves *et al.* (1996) and Cohen *et al.* (1996), and prospective studies reported by Tinker *et al.* (1997) and Kananee *et al.* (1997). Risk factors were identified by selecting factors that would increase the risk of colic. These researchers used logistic regression to statistically analyse and control confounding factors.

Cohort studies are regarded as the gold-standard of epidemiological study designs for measuring both the burden of illness (in terms of incidence and/or mortality) and in identifying risk factors (Rothman, 1986). The cohort study carried out by Tinker *et al.* (1997) involved selecting a population of horses on 31 farms in Virginia–Maryland that were initially free of disease, obtaining relevant information on possible risk factors, and then following the population prospectively through a period in which horses developing colic were recorded. The study showed that if 100 horses were followed for 1 year, 10 horses could be expected to show colic. These were predominantly simple colic cases with few strangulations, and therefore diseases related to age were not as prevalent. In a previous study that provided a valid measure of colic incidence, Uhlinger (1990), using a similar prospective cohort study on 12 horse farms in North Carolina, reported an incidence rate which varied between 19 and 39 colic cases per 100 horse years, substantially higher than the estimate from Virginia. A recent study in Michigan had a much lower incidence, at 3.5 colic episodes per 100 horse years. The much lower rate in this population remains unexplained (Kananee *et al.*, 1997). Knowing the incidence (and mortality) of a disease, even in a select population, is an important step forward in our knowledge because it helps us answer important practical questions such as, 'What rate of colic could we expect to see in this population?' (Reeves, 1997). Another notable finding from the Virginia–Maryland study was that the incidence of colic varied widely among the farms, from 0–30 cases per 100 horse years. Seven of the farms had incidence rates more than twice that of the overall study. Assuming the reporting was the same on each farm, these data suggest that there is a considerable amount of variability in colic incidence between different farms. In all likelihood, a combination of risk factors must be operating at the farm and individual horse level to cause such variability. If these factors could be identified, interventions could be sought to reduce colic incidence to a realistic minimum level.

Age, gender and breed

Age, gender and breed have been associated with increased risk of colic. Certain forms of colic appear to be more prevalent in younger animals (e.g. intussusceptions), while strangulating lipomas are a common cause of colic in old horses. Risk of colic was greatest for horses 2–10 years of age in the Virginia study, but this observation has not been corroborated by other studies. In one study, older horses appeared to require surgical management more frequently and to have a poorer prognosis for survival than young horses (Reeves *et al.*, 1989).

Some forms of colic are gender-specific (e.g. uterine torsion or inguinal hernia). Although not substantiated by an epidemiological study, colonic torsion appears to be more prevalent among mares. Gender has not been associated with colic as a general complaint.

Breed has been identified in a number of studies to be associated with increased risk of colic. The association may be related to differing management practices for Arabs, a greater concern about colic and its management by their owners, or a genetic predisposition to gastro-intestinal disorders among Arab horses. Certain breed predilections for specific types of colic have been suggested. Standardbreds appear to be at more of a risk of inguinal hernias than other breeds, and impactions and faecoliths of the small colon appear to be more prevalent in younger ponies.

Horses used for breeding have been reported to be at increased risk in several studies, but no specific factor associated with breeding (such as pregnancy, gestation or lactation) has been directly linked to the increased risk. Nutrition may be a confounder for use because horses used for breeding and strenuous sporting events are more likely to be fed a greater amount of concentrate to maintain weight and performance (White, 1997).

Geographic location or a particular environment can also be associated with increased risk of certain diseases. Enteroliths are seen only rarely in horses in Europe but are common in certain areas in the United States, where the incidence is highest in California, Florida and parts of the mid-west.

Other factors

Dental disorders are thought to predispose to certain forms of alimentary tract disease, such as choke and large colon impaction, but no association between colic and frequency of dental care has been reported. However, one study (Cohen *et al.*, 1996) found that more than 30 per cent of horses in a large population received dental care less than once yearly.

The evidence for parasitic control as a risk factor is limited and conflicting. Uhlinger (1990) concluded that parasites are an important cause of colic on some farms, that small strongyles are an important cause of parasitic colic, and that using control programmes to keep average faecal egg counts below 200 eggs/g will decrease the incidence of colic. Tinker *et al.* (1994) found no association between incidence of colic and the presence of strongyle eggs in the faeces. Reeves *et al.* (1996) reported a significantly decreased risk of colic for a small number of horses which had received pyrantel tartrate for at least 60 days during a 12-month period. In contrast, Cohen *et al.* (1996) found no association of colic with types of anthelmintic administered, whether they were rotated or whether there was history of recent (within 2 weeks) anthelmintic treatment. This study included 493 horses that had received pyrantel tartrate.

Weather changes are frequently associated with increased frequency of colic, but statistical proof of risk is largely lacking. Rollins and Clement (1979) observed an increased incidence of colic during the warmer months of the year. In contrast, Tinker *et al.* (1994) observed that most cases of colic in Virginia occurred in December and March, when the weather was relatively cool, and in August. Similar conflicting reports have been published relating to grass sickness (Edwards, 1995). Proudman (1991) found no association between colic and mean monthly temperature, mean monthly rainfall or mean monthly rainfall weighted for temperature. In the Virginia study (Tinker *et al.*, 1994), when events were investigated by looking at a 14-day window preceding colic episodes in both horses with colic and controls, low humidity marginally increased risk. No explanation for this relationship exists unless it is a confounder for management changes such as altering activity during weather extremes. A recent case–control study found an increased risk for weather changes, but the reliability of these observations by veterinarians was not confirmed.

History of previous colic

A history of previous colic has been identified repeatedly as a risk factor for colic (Cohen *et al.*, 1996; Kananee *et al.*, 1997; Reeves *et al.*, 1996 and Tinker *et al.*, 1997). Other studies have suggested that there is an increased risk after large colon impaction and surgery for abdominal disease. In some cases the reason for repeated colic is unclear, and proposed causes such as increased sensitivity to certain feeds or parasites have not been documented. It appears that some horses are simply more prone to colic, even under optimal management conditions (White, 1997). In order to determine a cause of disease, a factor or factors that significantly increases or decreases risk must first be identified and a significant reduction in incidence shown to occur when exposure to the factor is reduced. To date, only the first half of this requirement has been completed for risk factors reported for colic. Even so it is clear from the factors examined in all the studies that feeding and management factors are related to the frequency of colic. All the event factors point to management changes or factors that can influence physiologic changes and cause colic. Horses that are subject to change of activity or diet due to illness, medication administration or scheduling changes should be considered to be at increased risk of colic. Although individual horses may tolerate change with no problem, some are apparently more susceptible to intestinal dysfunction, and this may be sufficient to cause colic (White, 1997).

References

Abbott, E. M. (1998). Larval cyathostomosis. The disease, its diagnosis and treatment. *Equine Pract.*, **20(3)**, 6–7.

Adair, H. S. (1990). What is your diagnosis? *J. Am. Vet. Med. Assoc.*, **196**, 2023–4.

Argenzio, R. A. (1975). Functions of the equine large intestine and their inter-relationships in disease. *Cornel Vet.*, **65**, 303.

Argenzio, R. A. (1990). Physiology of digestive, secretory and absorptive processes. In *The Equine Acute Abdomen* (N. A. White, ed.), p. 23. Lea and Febiger.

Austin, S. M., Di Pietro, J. A., Foreman, J. H. *et al.* (1990). *Parascaris equorum* infections in horses. *Comp. Cont. Ed. Pract. Vet.*, **12(8)**, 1110–18.

Barclay, W. P., Phillips, T. W. and Foerner, J. J. (1982). Intussusception associated with *Anoplocephala perfoliata* infection in five horses. *J. Am. Vet. Med. Assoc.*, **180**, 752–3.

Beroza, G. A., Barclay, W. P. and Phillips, T. N. (1983). Caecal perforation and peritonitis associated with *Anoplocephala perfoliata* infection in three horses. *J. Am. Vet. Med. Assoc.*, **183**, 804–6.

Beroza, G. A., Barclay, W. P. and Phillips, T. N. (1986). Prevalence of tapeworm infection and associated large bowel disease in horses. *Proc. 2nd Equine Colic Res. Symp., Athens, Georgia*, **2**, 21–5.

Cable, C. S., Fubini, S. L., Erb, H. N. *et al.* (1996). Abdominal surgery in foals; a review of 119 cases (1977–1994). *Proc. ACVS*, 3.

Clarke, L. L., Williams, R. and Marcus, L. S. (1990). Feeding and digestive problems in horses. Physiological responses to a concentrated meal. *Vet. Clin. N. Am. Equine Pract.*, **6**, 433.

Clayton, H. M. and Duncan, J. L. (1979). Clinical signs associated with *Parascaris equorum* infection in worm-free ponies, foals and yearlings. *Vet. Parasitol.*, **4**, 69.

Clayton, H. M. (1986). Ascarids; Recent advances. *Vet. Clin. N. Am. Equine Pract.*, **2**, 313–28.

Cohen, N. B., Matejka, P. L., Honnas, C. M. *et al.* (1996). Case–control study of the association between various management factors and development of colic in horses. *J. Am. Vet. Med. Assoc.*, **206**, 667–73.

Cosgrove, J. S., Sheeran, J. J. and Sainty, T. J. (1986). Intussusception associated with infection with *Anoplocephala perfoliata* in a two-year-old thoroughbred. *Irish Vet. J.*, **40**, 35–6.

Dabareiner, D. M. and White, N. A. (1995). Large colon impaction in horses: 147 cases (1985–1991). *J. Am. Vet. Med. Assoc.*, **206**, 679–85.

Di Pietro, J. A. (1992). Internal parasite control programmes. In *Current Therapy in Equine Medicine* (N. E. Robinson, ed.), p. 3. W. B. Saunders Co.

Di Pietro, J. A. and Todd, K. S. (1988). Chemotherapeutic treatment of larvae and migratory stages of *Parascaris equorum*. *Proc. Ann. Conv. Am. Assoc. Equine Pract.*, **34**, 611–18.

Duncan, J. L. (1974). Field studies on the epidemiology of mixed strongyle infection in the horse. *Vet. Rec.*, **94**, 337–45.

Edwards, G. B. (1986). Intestinal diseases associated with *Anoplocephala perfoliata* in the horse. *Proc. 16th Cong. Eur. Soc. Vet. Surg., London*, pp. 99–105.

Edwards, G. B. (1995). Grass sickness – a surgeon's viewpoint. *Proceedings of the 1st International Workshop on Grass Sickness EMND and Related Disorders, Berne, Switzerland, 26th–27th October* (C. Hahn, V. Gerber, C. Herholz and I. G. Mayhew, eds), pp. 4–6.

Fogarty, V., Del Fiero, F. and Purnell, F. E. (1994). Incidence of *Anoplocephala perfoliata* in horses examined at an Irish abattoir. *Vet. Rec.*, **134**, 515–18.

Freeman, D. E. (1997). Overview of gastrointestinal physiology. *Proc. 5th Cong. Equine Med. Surg., Geneva, 14th–16th December*, pp. 15–21.

Gaugan, E. M. and Hackett, R. P. (1990). Intussusceptions in horses. 11 cases 1978–89. *J. Am. Vet. Med. Assoc.*, **1907,** 1373–5.

Georgi, J. R. (1973). The Kikuchi–Enigk model of *Strongylus vulgaris* migrations in the horse. *Cornel Vet.*, **63**, 220.

Haas, D. K. (1979). Equine parasitism. V.M SAC, **74**, 980–88.

Herd, R. P. (1987). New look at worm control. *Proc. Am. Assoc. Equine Pract.*, **33**, 55–65.

Kananee, J. B., Miller, R. A., Ross, W. A. *et al.* (1997). Risk factors for colic in Michigan equine population. *Prev. Vet. Med.*, **30**, 23–6.

Klei, T. R. (1997). Parasite control programmes. In *Current Therapy in Equine Medicine* (N. E. Robinson, ed.), p. 4. W.B. Saunders Co.

Love, S. (1997). Clinical aspects of equine intestinal parasitism. *Proc. 5th Cong. Equine Med. Surg., Geneva, 14th–16th December*, pp. 677–80.

Lyons, E. T., Drudge, J. H., Tolliver, S. C. and Swerczek, T. W. (1986). Pyrantel pamoate: Evaluating its activity against equine tapeworms. *Vet. Med.*, **81,** 280–85.

Mair, T. S. (1994). Outbreak of larval cyathostomosis in yearling and two-year-old horses. *Vet. Rec.*, **135,** 598–600.

Meyer, H. *et al.* (1993). Investigation on pre-ileal digestion of oats, corn and barley starch in relation to grain processing. *Proc. 13th Equine Nutr. Physiol. Symp.*

Ogbourne, C. P. (1971). Variations in the fecundity of strongylid worms of the horse. *Parasitology*, **63,** 289–98.

Owen, R. R., Jagger, D. W. and Quan-Taylor, R. (1989). Caecal intussusceptions in horses and the significance of *Anoplocephala perfoliata*. *Vet. Rec.*, **124,** 34–7.

Pagan, J. *et al.* (1997). Control colic through management. *World Equine Vet. Rev.*, **2,** 5.

Pearson, G. R., Davies, L. W. and White, A. C. (1993). Pathological lesions associated with *Anoplocephala perfoliata* at the ileocaecal junction of horses. *Vet. Rec.*, **132,** 179–82.

Pond, K. R. *et al.* (1993). Grazing behaviour of mares and steers on orchard grass and mares on common Bermuda grass. *Proc. 14th Equine Nutr. Physiol. Symp.*, p. 236.

Proudman, C. J. (1991). A two-year prospective study of equine colic in practice. *Equine Vet. J.*, **24,** 90.

Proudman, C. J. and Edwards, G. B. (1993). Are tapeworms associated with equine colic? A case–control study. *Equine Vet. J.*, **25,** 224–6.

Proudman, C. J. and Trees, A. J. (1996). Correlation of antigen specific IgG and IgG(T) responses with *Anoplocephala perfoliata* infection intensity in the horse. *Parasite Immunol.*, **18,** 499–506.

Proudman, C. J., French, N. P. and Trees, A. J. (1998). Tapeworm infection is a significant risk factor for spasmodic colic and ileal impaction colic in the horse. *Equine Vet. J.*, **30(3),** 194–9.

Reeves, J. J. (1997). What really causes colic in horses? Epidemiology's role in elucidating the ultimate multifactorial disease. *Equine Vet. J.*, **29(6),** 423–4.

Reeves, M. J., Curtis, C. R., Salman, M. D. *et al.* (1989). Prognosis in equine colic patients using multivariable analysis. *Can. J. Vet. Res.*, **53**, 87.

Reeves, M. J., Curtis, C. R., Salman, M. D. *et al.* (1996). Risk factors for equine acute abdominal disease (colic). Results from a multicentered case–control study. *Prev. Vet. Med.*, **26**, 285–301.

Reinemeyer, C. R. (1998). Practical and theoretical consequences of larvicidal therapy. *Equine Pract.*, **20(4)**, 10–17.

Rollins, J. B. and Clement, T. H. (1979). Observations on the incidence of equine colic in private practice. *Equine Pract.*, **1**, 39.

Rothman, K. L. (1986). *Modern Epidemiology*. Little Brown and Co.

Slocombe, J. O. D. (1979). Anthelmintic resistance in strongyles of equids. In *Equine Infectious Diseases. Proc. VI Int. Conf., Newmarket, England* (W. Plowright, P. R. Rossdale and J. P. Wade, eds), pp. 137–43. R & W Publications.

Slocombe, J. O. D. (1997). *Equine Infectious Diseases VI*, pp. 137–43. C. W. Publications.

Southwood, L. L., Ragle, C. A. and Snyder, J. (1996). Surgical treatment of ascariol impactions in horses and foals. *Proc. Ann. Conv. Am. Assoc. Equine Pract.*, **42**, 258–61.

Tinker, M. L., White, N. A., Lesard, P. *et al.* (1994). Descriptive epidemiology and incidence of colic on horse farms. A prospective study. *Proc. 5th Equine Colic Res. Symp., Athens, Georgia*, p. 22.

Tinker, M. K., White, N. A., Lessard, P. *et al.* (1997). Prospective study of equine colic risk factors. *Equine Vet. J.*, **29**, 454–8.

Uhlinger, C. A. and Brumbaugh, G. W. (1990). Parasite control programmes. In *Large Animal Internal Medicine* (B. M. Smith, ed.), pp. 1522–4. C. V. Mosby Co.

Uhlinger, C. (1990). Effects of three anthelmintic schedules on the incidence of colic in horses. *Equine Vet. J.*, **22**, 251–4.

Vasitas, N. J., Snyder, J. R., Wilson, W. D. *et al.* (1996). Surgical treatment for colic in the foal (67 cases); 1980–1992. *Equine Vet. J.*, **28**, 139–45.

White, N. A. (1981). Intestinal infarction associated with mesenteric vascular thrombotic disease in the horse. *J. Am. Vet. Med. Assoc.*, **178**, 259.

White, N. A. (1997). Risk factors associated with colic. In *Current Therapy in Equine Medicine* (N. E. Robinson, ed.), pp. 174–9. W. B. Saunders Co.

Index